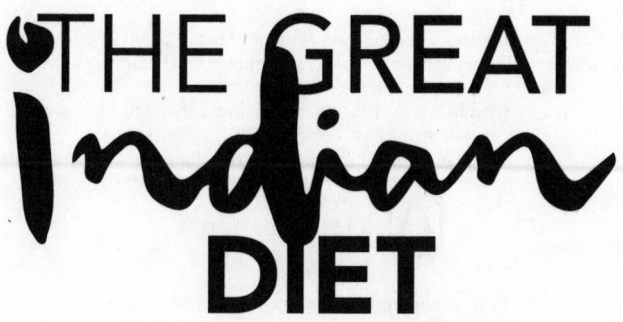

THE GREAT indian DIET

Busting the big **FAT MYTH**

D0968198

SHILPA SHETTY KUNDRA
LUKE COUTINHO

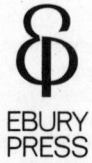

EBURY
PRESS

EBURY PRESS

USA | Canada | UK | Ireland | Australia
New Zealand | India | South Africa | China

Ebury Press is part of the Penguin Random House group of companies
whose addresses can be found at global.penguinrandomhouse.com

Published by Penguin Books India Pvt. Ltd
7th Floor, Infinity Tower C, DLF Cyber City,
Gurgaon 122 002, Haryana, India

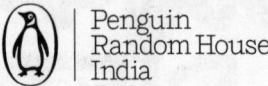

First published by Random House India 2015

ISBN 9788184007480

For sale in the Indian Subcontinent only

Typeset in Sabon by Manipal Digital Systems, Manipal
Printed at Thomson Press India Ltd, New Delhi

www.penguin.co.in

Nothing in life can be achieved without discipline and dedication, not even good health. I dedicate this book to all those people who care for their health and want to make it better. Those who don't (yet), I hope reading The Great Indian Diet *will show you how simple it is to lead a healthy life.*

And

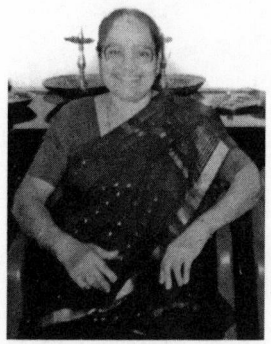

To the memory of Amma, my grandmother, who was the first to make me fall in love with Indian food.

Shilpa Shetty Kundra

*

I dedicate this book to my fellow Indians, and my family.

And

To Tyanna Brooklyn Coutinho, a reminder that life is 'priceless'.

Luke Coutinho

Contents

Foreword   vii
Preface   ix
Introduction   xvii

Part One: Indian Food

What Is the Great Indian Diet?   3
Is the Great Indian Diet Only a Diet to Lose Weight? 30

Part Two: What Is Going Wrong?

The Evils of the Food Industry   41
Foods That Are Bad for Health   46

Part Three: Understand What You Eat

The Components of a Healthy Meal   59
From Spices to Salt   81

Part Four: Lose Weight While You Eat Right

Understanding and Eliminating Fat   103
Lose Weight with the Great Indian Diet   111
The Great Indian Diet Plan   121

Part Five: Cook Healthy to Stay Healthy

Recipes for the Great Indian Diet 143
Chutneys, Papads and Pickles 159

Conclusion 169
Acknowledgements 175
Note on the Authors 179

Foreword

The Great Indian Diet by Shilpa Shetty Kundra and Luke Coutinho shows the path to healthy living and looking good by eating Indian food. In today's world, where everybody is running after the West for new ideas and trendy diets, this book comes as a welcome relief. It attempts to connect us back to our roots, things we have grown up eating, and shows us how we can use the knowledge already available to us to stay healthy and disease-free.

So what does health mean to me? It means the lifestyle choices that make us feel better, sleep better.

The choice of fuel we choose for our body is what can harm us, heal us or cause unnecessary stress to our bodies—inside and out.

This is Indian food, our food, our way. Follow the good old-fashioned beliefs. Eat the right food. Get a good nights' sleep and let your foods comfort, nourish and heal you. The right amount of good food can take us to the right destination. Read, enjoy, partake and relish what good food in right quantities can do for a healthy lifestyle.

I congratulate Shilpa and Luke on their brilliant effort and hope you all understand the importance of the great Indian diet. Let's all think global and eat local to stay fit, healthy and enjoy life to its fullest.

Anil Kapoor
Mumbai, August 2015

Preface

Hi! My name is Shilpa Shetty Kundra. Most of you know me as an actor, but I'm also a businesswoman, a fitness enthusiast, a wife and a full-time mother. My newest role, that of a 'health advocate', came about quite subconsciously through my journey of discovering motherhood. That made me realize the immense responsibility and role that food plays in making a life. I have always been complimented for my body and often been referred to as 'the body' (at the cost of being immodest), but most people don't know what goes into maintaining it. To be honest, I have never really paid too much attention to my body, but I value it and must have done something right to have remained at a constant 58 to 60 kilos for some twenty-two years.

Friends and fans generally think, 'What's the big deal? She's blessed with a great metabolism; she is born that way. Actors have it easy; they have money, which allows them access to the best trainers, nutritionists and supplements. You just have it without any hard work or effort.'

Here is the truth. Up to a point, maybe I believed it too. I just felt blessed to be endowed with good height and curves, but my health and my weight are completely the result of my habits, discipline and regime. I didn't truly value my body until I had my baby. It then struck me that I was only an ordinary woman who had the same fears, struggles and issues as any other woman.

I gained 32 kilos (yes, I was a whole new person and a half extra) during the pregnancy. The ideal Indian joint family I married into tried feeding me aloo parathas laced with white butter and gal gal ka achar (from Punjab, I had no idea something like that even existed, being south Indian), sarson da saag with makai di roti, and more white butter, and grated jaggery. I enjoyed those, to be honest, and I'm not complaining.

By the way, three kilos came from the halwa Bijee made for me every second day while I was carrying Viaan, which I ate with no regrets. Today the family discusses grilled foods and boiled sprouts. I think it is the 'SSK effect'. You can't beat 'em, join 'em! Getting back in shape was quite a difficult and challenging journey. It was frustrating, dealing with all that extra weight, an alteration in body image and all the changes that pregnancy brings along with it. To confess, I did let go during that time. I thought I would do everything the old-fashioned way, and so I ate and put on more weight than I should have. After Viaan Raj (my son) was born, I wanted my body back really badly, not just for the sake of looks, but because I felt unhealthy. I did not feel like my natural self on the inside or the outside. Seven months after the delivery, I decided to get my health back on track. I lost 28 kilos in four months, and believe me, it was far from easy.

It was difficult, but not impossible, and that's the way it will always be. The day you set your mind to a goal and decide to achieve it, you will see the change begin to happen.

Any weight loss regime, I assure you, is 70 per cent diet and 30 per cent exercise, coupled with good sleep and a positive frame of mind. I believe it's all in the mind; it's mind over body because that is where it starts. I had a vision of how I wanted to look and feel in my mind, and I worked only towards that. I refused to be blinded or confused by the theories, fad diets and exercise programmes that the media, magazines or social groups advocate. I had a vision firmly formed in my mind, and I just set out to achieve it.

What is my secret?

I don't diet. Yes, it is true. The word 'diet' makes the mind believe that the body is being deprived, and this deprivation leads to cravings. Sample this. During karva chauth fasts, I start to crave all kinds of things. It's all in the mind. I have never believed in diets and never will, but what I live by is a healthy regime, good food, real food—or what Luke and I call 'the Great Indian Diet'—adequate exercise that suits my body and restful sleep. I use yoga and meditation to manage any stress and stay positive in every situation. I also believe that it's important to understand the type of body you have. Ayurveda defines this in the best way possible. For example, if your constitution is vata, pitta or kapha, there will be certain foods that suit you and some that won't, and it's important to know this.

With my erratic schedules, sometimes I don't exercise for several weeks, but I balance it out with food to ensure that I don't put on weight. That's a choice we all have, and it's a great choice. Moderation and compensation in all ways to achieve a healthy and happy lifestyle is what works.

No matter what obstacles you face in your journey to weight loss or better health, stay positive. Negativity will drag you down. Pick yourself up and move on.

Why this book?

My journey through shedding my baby fat happened in full public view as I was shooting for a dance reality show at the time. People, friends, my stylist, everybody saw me drop weight, inches and dress sizes on a weekly basis, much to their surprise. By the end of seven weeks, I was lighter by 32 kilos. Everyone wanted to know my exercise regimen and what I was eating (or not). Some secretly believed liposuction was the secret behind my weight loss.

I won't deny briefly thinking of it as a last option, when I looked at myself in the mirror seven months after my son was born. I realized I had let myself go and thought I'd never be able to be my old svelte self again! (For an actor, vanity comes with the package, but honesty doesn't!) But I don't like things easy.

What I also realized was that everyone around me, including myself at the time, was 'weight obsessed' rather than 'health obsessed'. It made me wonder if that equation would ever change. We seriously need to change our perspective on that first. Despite belonging to the beauty business, I've always emphasized that health comes first!

The last three years, in my own small way, I have also been encouraging people I am close to, to make small changes in their eating habits and timings. Starting with relatives, I have often lectured my sister-in-law Reena, who lives in the UK, about throwing out all sugar-laden cereals and foods with artificial colours and preservatives, and monitoring my nieces' intake of fizzy drinks. She has sweetly obliged out of love, or perhaps just to get me to stop telling her about the mental and physical side-effects they have in the future. Not that she didn't care, but she didn't know any better. She, like most of us, is a working mother.

I understand that a lot of us tend to get over-indulgent. The first cause is that when we are back from work, mostly exhausted, we want to take it easy and so given in to our children's demands. Another cause is that it is hard to constantly keep an eye on them and become a nag. It is a hard, thankless job but someone's got to do it! Discipline is key and that's also my favourite word, as you will realize when you read through the book.

Reena has seen the difference the small changes have made in her children's lives and health. She is thankful today and that's all that matters. I think if I can play a catalyst in a few people's lives, my purpose on earth (without being dramatic) would have been fulfilled. This is my calling.

While all this sounded great, it dawned upon me that I can't do this on my own. I needed someone who shared the same vision and passion about Indian food as I. Someone who belonged to this milieu, to illustrate my thoughts with experience and experiments. And I found that person in Luke Coutinho.

I met Luke Coutinho, an acclaimed nutritionist, author, cancer specialist, speaker and fitness consultant, through a common friend who recommended him to me to help with a nutrition plan for my son.

I remember the first time I met Luke. I said, 'You look like a school boy; I was expecting someone older.' From then on, it's been an exciting journey, filled with a lot of learning, great ideas, memorable experiences and conversations. I had thoughts and he reiterated my beliefs with proof in surveys.

Luke and I are alike in so many ways. We have met more often as friends to discuss nutrition, eating habits, lifestyle, exercise, new fads, diseases and latest juice concoctions. We both don't believe in diets and are in complete sync about how making small changes in lifestyle is sustainable, long-lasting and the way forward.

We discovered similar likes and passions, and talked about new ideas to help people become healthier. he witnessed me shrink from 83 kilos to 58 kilos and saw Viaan grow up into a healthy young boy. We had the same thoughts and he backed it with knowledge and surveys. I'm so glad he helped me decode nutrition and demystify health and lifestyle. The most important thing we have in common is our dream to see people proud of our food— the Indian diet—and use it to get healthier. We want to make people aware that it's not just food, exercise and sleep, but also your mind-body connection that is responsible for great health, well-being and happiness.

I can't thank you enough, Luke, for being a part of my journey, to good health as well as of writing *The Great Indian Diet*. This book has been a learning curve, even for me.

Meeting Luke was destiny, not planned, and that makes me believe that this book was predestined to happen. As Luke and I believe, every Indian and world citizen should own this book, because we believe and intend for it to change lives and health across the globe in the simplest way possible.

Shilpa Shetty Kundra

Introduction

My interest in nutrition began in college. Since then, I haven't looked back, following up with certifications from Australia and New York. now, my sessions on nutrition, forming nutrition plans, and work with Yale, take me all around the world.

I remember I was in Goa, back home with my family, when Shilpa called me and asked to meet up to discuss nutrition once I was back in Mumbai. On that very call, I remember how we both got talking for quite some time about nutrition and lifestyle.

What impressed me the most about Shilpa during my first visit was her humility, her willingness to listen and learn, her curiosity, her passion about health, lifestyle and nutrition, and the fact that she is a hands-on mom who does everything herself and is completely involved in Viaan's day-to-day activities, food, routine and well-being.

All through her pregnancy and even after it, Shilpa used commonly available Indian spices and preparations. Viaan's food plan was also completely based on nutritious Indian food.

It's been almost three years since I have known Shilpa. I saw her transform from 83 kilos to 58 kilos through sheer dedication, will power and without any crazy exercise or diet plan. She used no supplements, protein shakes or fad food, and the plan she followed was far from restrictive. There was quite a bit to eat, but it was wholesome food with generous amounts of homemade ghee and limited amounts of sugar. The exercise regimen she stuck to was something she enjoyed and followed in a controlled manner. There was no over-exercising. More than anything, it was her positive outlook and attitude that got her to 58 kilos in a healthy way. What impressed me the most about Shilpa was the fact that there were no excuses, complaints or blame, something that most people struggling to lose weight or get fit tend to wallow in. She knew she hadn't exercised restraint. She was aware of the reason she had put on the extra kilos and knew exactly what she had to do to get back in shape, and she did just that. There was no looking for short-cuts, no complaining about how tough it was or blaming it on hormones, motherhood, being a woman, etc. She simply did it using common sense and simplicity, powered by passion and the right attitude. In this book, we are going to share the exact plans that were created by her sensibilities to which was added my expertise to make a foolproof diet plan, to show everyone that weight loss is far from difficult and that restrictive diets and crazy exercise programmes don't work.

Shilpa and I share the same passions, thoughts and ideas when it comes to health. I remember going over all the food plans she created for her friends and family members, her most recent success being a superb plan for her father-in-law who suffered from gout. Balkrishna Kundra lost 13 kilos in six weeks and also brought about a change in his lifestyle.

Two years ago, Shilpa and I were on a long flight, heading back to India. As usual, we started talking about our favourite subject—health and nutrition. What began with sharing notes and discussing food plans soon shifted to some of the latest research that the medical and nutrition world has been working on for many years, i.e. spices, different kinds of food, macronutrients, vitamins, minerals, antioxidants, herbs, etc. and then it struck us that most of the food, herbs and spices grow in our own country, India. We have an abundance of the very food that universities and research centres across the world are currently studying.

Shilpa asked me to pull out some of the notes and plans that I had compiled, and we realized that if we could fit in at least 80 per cent Indian foods and spices, or maybe even 90 per cent, we would achieve a near-perfect food plan.

What were these Indian foods, spices, herbs, beverages, nuts and seeds that could prevent and maybe even cure the deadliest of diseases, help burn fat, improve energy levels, detoxify the liver, colon and blood, and boost immunity? It was then that we realized how blessed we were. We lived in a country where we had access to some of the most nutritious food in the world. In fact, most countries across the world now have access to Indian food, thanks to technology and advanced logistics. We have everything in our own country, and if used in the right way, it can prevent and cure diseases, and possibly alter the country's health statistics.

For many years, we were completely convinced that the Mediterranean diet with its staples of fruits, vegetables whole grains legumes and nuts indigenous to the region was the healthiest in the world. It is healthy; there is no doubt about that, but when Shilpa and I decided to break it down in detail and compare it with the Indian diet, we began to believe, and are now completely convinced, that the Indian diet is as healthy, or might we say, even healthier than the Mediterranean diet.

Every country or region will have its own diet that is local and healthy for the people that live there. The Mediterranean diet will perhaps be healthy for people living in the Mediterranean region, like the Chinese diet would be healthy for those in China. In fact, there is a lot of extremely healthy food that is common to almost all cuisines globally.

On that flight, Shilpa and I decided to write this book with the intent to change the health and lives of people in India and across the world in the simplest way possible. We studied the Indian diet in detail and put it all together with the help of research teams, renowned doctors and nutritionists across the globe.

This is not just a book. It's the beginning of a journey. Through it, we intend to give India and the world a solution to this weight and disease epidemic, and the best part of the solution is that it does not have anything to do with dieting.

We reiterate that the best diet according to us is the Indian diet when it comes to losing weight, gaining weight, building greater immunity, and even preventing or curing diseases.

During this journey, we have worked with people across the globe from all fields that have used Indian food or parts of the Indian diet to change their health for the better. We began to educate people outside India about the amazing benefits of Indian food, and most people quickly embraced it, or some parts of it, to change their health. We began working on plans that incorporated grains, spices, herbs and other food from Indian cuisine into food plans and continued to reap positive benefits. Most importantly, people were beginning to enjoy this change.

Why should you read this book?

It will open your eyes to the beauty, power and amazing nutrition of the food already around you, food that you have probably consumed for years, but maybe not in the right quantities, combinations and patterns.

We want to inspire leaders, politicians, children, parents, schools, teachers, models and actors to embrace healthy food and lifestyles. We want people to understand and respect the power of food and what nature has gifted us. We can reduce suffering and death caused by many diseases if we change our lifestyles and the way we eat.

It is our desire to inspire people to believe that great food can cure, prevent and heal deadly diseases and enrich lifestyles and health.

We want to dispel myths about Indian food, fats, sugars, and everything there is to do with the Indian diet.

We want people to know that you can get more than sufficient protein in the Indian diet, and you do not have to compromise your religion or beliefs by switching to eggs or meat if you are a vegetarian.

We want people to understand all about Vitamin B_{12} and Vitamin D_3, and how an Indian diet and a healthy lifestyle is more than sufficient to maintain healthy levels of these crucial vitamins.

We want people to know that the two important tools are moderation and compensation, and that it's alright to enjoy your life and the food you eat.

We want people to be proud of the Indian diet and not be deceived or programmed by media, movies, magazines, etc., which divert them from the diet staples. Should we fall prey to advertisements for 'weight loss pills', 'fat-free food', 'health bars', and the protein craze? It is our desire to make people realize that simplicity wins in all aspects of life, including your body and health.

It breaks our hearts when a lover of Indian food is told to switch to other food, like quinoa, chia seeds, blueberries and so on—the very food that is *not local* to India—for health or weight loss reasons. People are asked to give up pure farm ghee and switch to processed oils.

We mean no disrespect to this global food; it is extremely healthy, but why should it replace our staple diet of brown rice, Indian millets, flaxseeds, local fruits and vegetables? Why should olive oil replace the traditional Indian mustard, groundnut, coconut, sunflower, rice bran oils or pure ghee?

Health Tourism

On a skiing holiday with actor Madhavan, we got talking about his health and weight. Madhavan loves his food and had put on some extra weight when he had to stop working out because of a nagging knee ailment. As a friend, I encouraged him to start looking at his overall health. He made a visit to a famous health camp in Austria and on returning, shared with me what the head nutritionist there told him. His advice was that Madhavan should go back to India after the camp and consume the traditional Indian diet. How ironic that he, being a European, would encourage Indians to go back to their country and consume Indian food for good health.

Madhavan swears by the statement 'chew your water and drink your food', and it's simple lifestyle changes and dedication to the great Indian diet that keeps him fit and healthy.

Working with doctors, oncologists and surgeons across the globe, it is important to mention how most post-recovery plans I make include Indian food and spices. I completely believe that food can be your medicine in most cases.

The Power of the Mind

Are you aware of this free drug that can help treat many disorders, weight problems, diseases and other conditions with no side-effects? Yes, it is our mind. The power of the mind is one of the strongest and most useful powers you possess. This power consists of your thoughts.

In my experience with cancer patients worldwide, I have seen amazing transformations that can take place when they start believing and using their minds to heal.

If you think you are fat, you will be fat. If you think you are sick, you will be sick. Manifesting a disease is real. I know a lady who manifested cancer as she was told by several fortunetellers that at a particular age she would suffer from cancer. She kept believing that it would happen, and lived in constant fear. Eventually, she did get cancer.

The thoughts that pass through your mind are responsible for what happens in your body. Your predominant thoughts influence your behaviour and attitude, and control your actions and reactions. The best part is that you can train and strengthen this power. You can use it to make changes in your life and influence other peoples' minds.

If you plant seeds, water them and give them fertilizers, they will grow into healthy and strong plants. Thoughts, like seeds, have a natural tendency to grow and manifest in your life if you feed them with attention, interest and enthusiasm.

The power of your mind is part of the creative power of the universe, which means that your thoughts work together with it. You are a manifestation of the universal mind.

When you repeat the same thought over and over again, in one way or another, this mighty power helps you make your thoughts come true. Pay attention to the thoughts you think. Do your best to reject negative thoughts and to allow into your mind only thoughts that bring good, happy and positive results.

If you really want to be healthy, first believe in your mind that you are. If you want to lose weight or heal, first believe that you can.

Dieting vs Lifestyle Changes

Diets don't work. Lifestyle changes do, coupled with smart exercising that you enjoy, restful sleep, effective management of stress, good, enjoyable and wholesome food, and belief in the power of your mind. That's our concept. I believe workouts should be over in thirty minutes, and we should enjoy what we eat completely and feel no guilt even if it's something not very healthy. We believe that incorporating meditation into our lives completes the whole equation of meaningful living.

People should not use exercise as a punishment for over-eating. We need to find a balance between all the aspects that contribute to a happy and healthy life. Over the years, my work has led me to believe that we need a fundamentally different way of looking at healthcare. We need a system that works beyond simply just looking at the symptoms that bring people into clinics, and instead be able to look at where health begins— not within the four walls of a doctor's clinic or a hospital, but where we live, work, eat, sleep, learn and play.

We may be living in a polluted world with pesticide-laden food, water that we think is clean and pure but may not be, air that consists of several deadly carcinogens, cosmetics and hair colours laden with chemicals, toxic junk food, etc. The list is endless.

How do we react to this? We keep running around, like headless chickens, searching for the next best healthy option and getting sucked into fads, diet programmes and dangerous exercise regimens.

Stop, step back and slow down. The answer to disease prevention and cure is *immunity*. It is your body's first and last line of defence against all health issues.

The foundation of what I do is absolute reverence, respect, and awe of nature. We get everything that is good for our body, mind and health from nature, and we were not designed to fall apart and fall sick as often as we do today.

Our practice now focuses on prevention, cure, healing and enhancing health. We look at disease or illness as a divine touch on the shoulder.

What we hope to achieve is to remind people that we are all products of nature, and therefore, we respond to the biological parameters that define us, i.e., nature. So, if we are able to align our lives, which include the way we eat, sleep, move and think, with nature, we will naturally thrive. Then, anything that's a problem, whether we call it arthritis, heart disease, obesity, weight gain or cancer, goes away because our body is a product of nature, and it is designed to heal itself if we allow it to, and if we keep it aligned with nature.

We don't fight disease, we support health, for where there is health, there is peace and where there is peace, there is healing.

We want people to know that there are hundreds of different diseases, which implies hundreds of different causes and possibly a hundred different cures. So, we should not restrict ourselves to just one line of treatment or belief and leverage the healing power of our bodies.

What is required to restore health is the same thing that is required to maintain health; healing or treatment aligned with nature.

We stopped believing in diets a long time ago. The concept of restrictive diets never impressed us, nor did it work for most people (in some cases, however, restrictive diets are necessary because of medical complications). A restrictive diet is one in which you stop eating a particular food component, like carbohydrate or proteins.

Restrictive diets lead to nutritional deficiencies, rapid and unhealthy weight loss, and in many cases, frustration and depression. People who commit to these diets age faster, look and feel awful, and almost always regain all the lost weight (and many times even more) after going back to a normal food plan. These diets focus just on weight and never really on fat loss or overall health. People drive themselves silly just to fit into that dress or get that body for an upcoming holiday or wedding. In the process, they lose out on much more.

If there's any one solid solution we have found in all the years of our experience, travels, studies and interactions, it's making a lifestyle change. Making a lifestyle change when it comes to your health and well-being brings about greater benefits than you could possibly imagine. It's magical, sustainable and motivating. It changes the way you think and behave, and it teaches you to respect your body. Diets don't work; if you want to lose weight and keep it off, you have to make a lifestyle change. But what does a lifestyle change look or feel like, and how do you know when you've made one?

The basic difference between a diet mentality and a lifestyle mentality is simply a matter of perspective.

- A diet is all about numbers—the number on the scale and the number of calories you eat and burn. Success is defined in terms of how well you stick to your numbers. A lifestyle change is all about you. It's about lining up your eating and physical activity with your real goals and desires. Success is defined in terms of how these changes make you feel about yourself.

- The diet mentality assumes that reaching a certain weight is the key to finding happiness and solving other problems. The lifestyle approach assumes that being overweight is usually the result of other problems, not the cause.
- Going on a diet involves an external and temporary change in your eating technique. You start counting and measuring, and you stop eating some foods and substitute others, based on the rules of whatever diet plan you are using. The results of a diet are external; if you're lucky, you may change on the outside but not on the inside.

Making a lifestyle change involves an internal and permanent change in your relationship with food, eating and physical activity. You recognize that the primary problem isn't what you eat or even how much you eat, but how and why you eat. Eating mindlessly and impulsively (without intention or awareness) and using food to manage your emotions and distract yourself from unpleasant thoughts is what really needs to change.

We hope this book will take you through a journey of great Indian food and at the end of it, you will be equipped to build your own personal food plan for yourself or your family. It's really simple when you are clearly aware of your goal, and you couple that with knowledge, a dose of discipline, and the right attitude to achieve the body and health you want. Come, be a part of this journey with us and discover the Great Indian Diet.

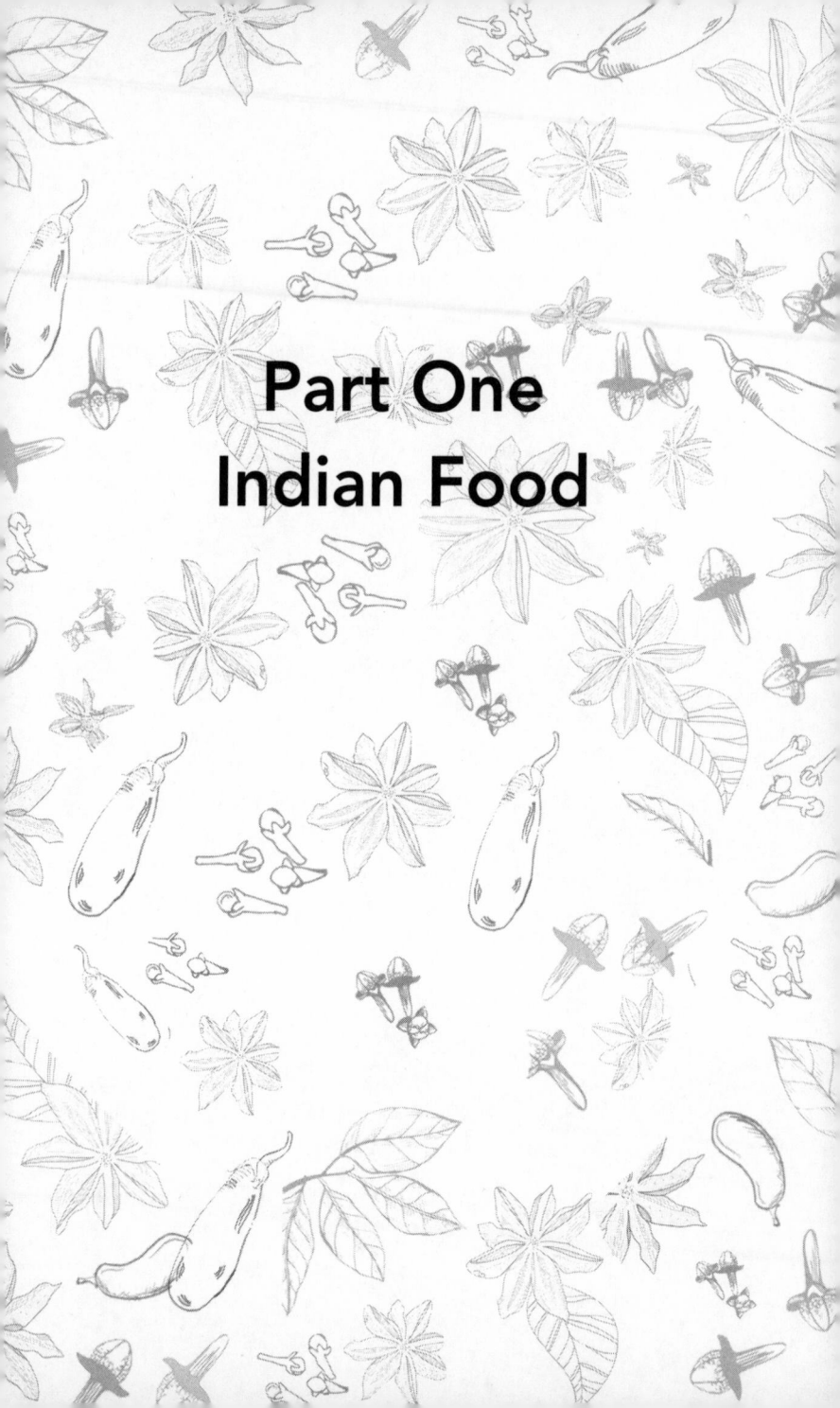

Part One
Indian Food

What Is the Great Indian Diet?

Come on, be honest. What are the first things that come to your mind when you think of Indian food? Hot, spicy, oily, rich, fatty, difficult and time-consuming to cook, something that has curry powder and sugar, and involves deep frying? You could say any of the above if the food was badly prepared or used the wrong way, and it is true of any other cuisine! Indian food, though hugely popular, is highly misunderstood. Several lifetimes are not enough to discover and sample all the delights of Indian cuisine. It is the glorious result of thousands of years of evolution and assimilation. Like all things Indian, food too has absorbed various influences from other cultures but has managed to make them uniquely its own. It is exotic, healthy, nutritious and sometimes complex, but always delicious.

Evolution of Indian Food

Indian cuisine has a history that is as old as that of civilization on the subcontinent—a period that spans five thousand years. It has developed as a result of various cultures that interacted with each other here, leading to the culinary richness we see in India today. The ancient medicinal and dietary science of Ayurveda classified food according to its qualities – Sattvic or pure foods, Rajasic or rich and stimulating foods, and Tamasic or heavy and difficult-to-digest foods. Indian diet has invariably been a combination of these, comprising fruit, vegetables, grains, eggs, milk and dairy products, honey, and sometimes meat. Over time, vegetarianism came to be adopted, especially during the ascendancy of religious movements like Buddhism and Jainism. A vegetarian diet in India is made feasible by its equitable climate that allows for a wide variety of fruit, vegetables and grains to be grown here in all seasons.

During the Middle ages, travellers to India introduced new cooking methods and products to the region, including tea and spices. North India was later invaded by Central Asian cultures, which led to the emergence of Mughlai cuisine, a mix of Indian and Central Asian cuisine. Hallmarks of this influence include the use of seasonings such as saffron.

Historical incidents, such as foreign invasions, trade relations and colonialism, have played an important role in introducing certain foods to the country. For instance, potato—now a staple of Indian diet—was brought to India by the Portuguese, who also introduced chilly and breadfruit. There has also been a Central Asian influence on North Indian cuisine from the years of Mughal and Turkic Delhi Sultanate rule. Similarly, Indian cuisine has also shaped the history of international relations; the spice trade between India and Europe is often cited by historians as the primary catalyst for Europe's Age of Discovery. Spices were bought from India and traded across Europe and Asia. It also influenced other cuisines across the world, especially those from Southeast Asia, the British Isles and the Caribbean. The evolution of these cuisines has been at times shaped by religious beliefs and in particular by vegetarianism, which is a growing dietary trend in Indian society. Indian cuisine has been and is still evolving, as a result of the nation's cultural interactions with other societies.

India's range of cuisines can amaze even a connoisseur. Different regions in India offer their own specialties with their unique taste, subtlety and aroma. The exotic tastes, hues, nutrition and textures of the Indian diet have found a steady acceptance and growth in popularity in Western countries. Its combination of fresh ingredients and gastronomic delight fulfil today's requirements for healthy eating. The great Indian diet surprises us with its incomparable flavours and scents, thanks to the use of specific combinations of spices.

The Main Components of Indian Food

India is known for its varied, spicy and delicious food. It is renowned not only for its taste but also its aroma. From your house you can identify what is being cooked at your neighbour's, just by the aroma of the dish. The reason for this is the use of spices in each recipe. Most Indian homes store spices for the whole year, the most common being rai (mustard seeds), haldi (turmeric), dalchini (cinnamon), elaichi (cardamom), lavang (cloves), jeera (cumin), bay leaves, tamarind, kokum, red chillies, fenugreek seeds and coriander powder. Ingredients like garlic, ginger, curry leaves, coconut, and many others, are used fresh. Each state of the country has its own pre-mixed blend of spices known as 'garam masala', which is used in dishes every day. Around the country, you will find unique blends of the above-mentioned spices, such as goda masala for Maharashtrian dishes, sambhar masala for South Indian food, biryani masala for a Hyderabadi flavour, chhole masala for Punjabi food, and so on.

Another important aspect of cooking is the medium which the food is cooked in, and which imparts an additional taste to all recipes. Oil or ghee is often the first ingredient that goes into the cooking vessel and is essential to the making of a delicious dish. The use of oil differs from state to state based on region, culture and climate. In North India, for instance, mustard oil is popular, while groundnut and sunflower oils are used for daily cooking in West India. Sesame oil imparts flavour to East Indian food, while in South India the staple cooking medium is coconut oil.

Some recipes demand the use of ghee, particularly sweets like sheera and various types of ladoos. Hydrogenated vegetable oil, known as 'dalda', is another popular cooking medium. It is losing its popularity, though, because research has shown its harmful effects on health.

Milk and milk products, like curd, buttermilk, cream, cheese and paneer, are widely used throughout India. Milk, cream, and sometimes even curd, are used in vegetable gravies, curries, rice preparations and in desserts.

The staples of all kinds of Indian cuisine are cereals like wheat, bajra, jowar, maize, ragi, as well as pulses like rajma, chhole, moong, matki, chawli (chickpea), as well as vegetables, fruits, nuts and seeds.

There is wide variety in Indian food which is influenced by religion, culture, climate and geographical location. The taste, colour, texture and cooking methods of Indian food change according to the region you are in, but its main components remain almost the same – cereals, pulses, fruits, vegetables, spices, fats, nuts and oilseeds.

Indian food has evolved over thousands of years and is the ultimate symbol of how Indian culture has the ability to absorb other influences, yet hold its own.

Did You Know?

- A traditional Indian meal is completely balanced as it includes all the food groups and nutrients required for healthy nutrition. It takes care of both macro as well as micro nutrients with the inclusion of carbohydrates (roti, rice, bhakhri etc.), proteins (non-vegetarian food, milk and milk products, pulses and legumes), fats (oils, ghee, nuts and seeds), fibre, vitamins and minerals (fruits and vegetables).

- Indian cooking involves the daily use of certain spices like turmeric, cumin, mustard seeds, heeng (asafoetida), ginger, garlic and green chillies, all of which have medicinal properties. Their use ensures that our body remains protected in all seasons.

- Any Indian woman can create her own recipe book due to the vast array of recipes that she has access to, each with a perfect blend of healthy nutrients in the form of seasonal fruits and vegetables, cereals, pulses, milk and milk products, and nuts.

- Indians have a tradition of cooking fresh food every day. Due to this, the use of preservatives is avoided to a large extent.
- Indian food has six tastes—sweet, salty, bitter, sour, astringent, and spicy. These ensure that people get all the nutrients through their food.

Myths about Indian Food

1. All Indian food is hot and spicy

Before we jump to this conclusion, we need to understand the difference between 'hot' and 'spicy'. The green or red chillies are what make food hot, while its spiciness is due to the spices used, like bay leaves, cinnamon, cloves, and so on. The veins and seeds of chillies contain a compound known as capsaicin, which is responsible for its hot taste, and can be detrimental when consumed in excess. The food which Indians prepare at home daily makes limited use of chillies and spices, which actually help maintain a healthy life due to the high level of antioxidants present in them.

In fact, I would say that with the use of chillies and spices, not-so-loved vegetables like spinach, bitter gourd and bottle gourd can also be made palatable and tasty. The thumb rule is to use spices and chillies in appropriate quantities.

2. Indian food is fattening and unhealthy

Excess of anything is bad for one's health. Eating too much of something that is deemed healthy will harm your health, since over-eating is known to store the extra food as fat in the body. Hence, I feel the above statement is applicable to any type of food, not just Indian food.

While cooking at home, one is mindful of things like the type and amount of oil used. One ensures that oil once used is not reused for frying or cooking, a practice that causes oxidation of oil, thereby rendering it harmful to the body.

Food served in a restaurant, or when prepared for special occasions, can be fattening and unhealthy since health is compromised in the interest of taste. In order to make it tastier than normal, many ingredients are used in excess—oil, butter, cream, sugar, and so on. When we go out to eat, few restaurants serve whole wheat rotis and so we end up eating unhealthy naans or roomali rotis which are made with refined wheat flour. We also tend to smear them with butter, while at home we would have done so with ghee, which is 'good fat' and helps in weight loss.

3. Indian gravies are unhealthy

I would agree if these gravies and curries are cooked with lots of oil, cream, cashewnuts and cheese. I make regular curries and gravies at home but their base is prepared with onion, tomato, ginger, garlic, coconut, yoghurt, besan, and garam masala. This is the common practice in most Indian homes. Some gravies call for specific ingredients like peanuts, dals, curry leaves, adding which is also a healthy option.

Healthy Curry

Alternative option for onion-based gravies is to pre-roast the onions with a teaspoon of coconut oil or vegetable oil in the grill, or an air-frier. You can mash the onions or add them as they are to the remaining mixture.

When curries and gravies are made on special occasions, we do tend to make them differently, with more oil, cream and so on, which is unhealthy.

'As a biochemist and nutritionist, I feel that the Indian thali is a role model for virtuous nutrition. I would say what makes it unique is the spices that we add to it. One of the most important spices that makes an Indian thali wholesome according to me is garlic. Taking into account the biochemical perspective, it has an action of inhibiting the enzymes of lipid mechanism, which is what makes it more powerful. Therefore, a simple garlic clove can help in reducing bad cholesterol and is anti-inflammatory. Garlic is very heart-friendly and relieves a simple cold too. A few chopped raw garlic pieces would definitely help improve our immunity as it is easy for everyone to add to soups or salads. Being full of antioxidants, it also helps in fighting cancer. Hang in there, because it is very important to have it in raw form, else you will destroy the allicin in it and its benefits.'
Manisha Guram, Biochemist, Nutrition – GOQii

What Makes the Indian Diet Healthy?

One thing you will observe about many Indian women is their possessiveness about their kitchens. I used to wonder why my mother didn't like anyone entering her kitchen or messing it up. When I got married, I saw my mother-in-law behave in the same way. I got the answer only after I took charge of my own kitchen. For a woman, the kitchen is where she takes care of her family's health. Peep into the kitchen of any Indian home, and you will find it crowded but well-maintained. You will see all the food groups nicely arranged on the shelves, like cereals, pulses, oils, nuts, milk and milk products, fruits, vegetables and eggs. This shows what makes Indian food healthy—the presence of all the food groups that a person requires for a healthy diet.

So far, we have discussed only individual food groups, but what is truly remarkable about Indian cuisine are the nutritious recipes which are prepared using combinations of food groups. If you have visited restaurants that serve 'thali', you will know of the kind of variety that exists in Indian food. Every state has its own thali, but its composition is somewhat similar. It typically includes:

- Roti, bhakhri, puri, idli or dosa, rice, khichadi (cereals—carbohydrates)
- Dal, rasam, sambhar, usal (pulses, beans, legumes—proteins)
- Dry and curried sabzi (seasonal vegetables—fibre, vitamins, minerals)
- Paneer sabzi, yoghurt, buttermilk (milk and milk products—proteins, calcium)
- Raita (yoghurt, vegetables)

- Chutney made of coconut, coriander, mint, peanuts, flaxseeds, garlic
- Dessert (milk and milk products, sugar, jaggery, honey)

Let's take a quick look at individual constituents of the thali and their wonderful traits:

Roti, chapati, bhakhri

These are made with wheat flour, to which are added oil, salt and water. The ingredients are mixed well to prepare the dough. Small balls of the dough are then flattened with a rolling pin and roasted on a heated pan to make hot and fluffy chapatis, which are an excellent source of carbohydrates. Indians also consume rotis made of bajra and jowar, grains that have a higher content of fibre. An important feature of bajra, jowar, and makai rotis is you do not require oil to make their dough. Nowadays people mix two or three cereals, like wheat with soya, to make the flour more nutritious.

Rice

Rice is a staple food in southern India, Assam and Kashmir. It is rich in starch, moderate in proteins and poor in fat, iron and calcium. Parboiled rice is a healthier version of white rice. In it, the vitamins and minerals from the bran get absorbed into the kernel, hence the nutrition of the whole grain is not lost when it is processed.

Switch to Brown

Brown rice is the healthiest form of rice, because it retains the inner seed coating called rice bran, and provides additional dietary fibre, vitamins, minerals and proteins. These days brown rice is in the limelight due to its high nutritional content. Switch from white to brown, brown rice, jaggery or brown sugar, and brown bread for good health.

Rice is simple to cook. Just take the required amount of rice, add double the amount of water, and pressure cook it.

A variety of healthy dishes can be prepared by combining rice with vegetables, garlic, ginger and spices, to impart aroma, flavour and additional nutrition to it.

Pulses and Lentils

Pulses, lentils, beans like rajma (kidney beans), matki (moth), chawli (chickpeas), brown chana, whole green gram (moong), and so on provide protein, complex carbohydrates, and several vitamins and minerals. Iron, magnesium, phosphorus, zinc and other minerals, which play a variety of roles in maintaining good health, are also present in them. Most curry recipes are prepared with the above-mentioned foods, which require more oil and cream to make them tasty. But they can be made healthy by using spices, curd and milk, instead of oil and cream.

Lentils can be boiled with tomatoes, rock salt and tempered with only a spoon of ghee, curry leaves, jeera, hing and dry whole red chillies. Garnish with coriander and serve hot. How's that fattening or unhealthy?

Vegetables

Vegetables are extensively used in Indian cuisine. Low in calories, high in fibre, minerals and vitamins, they are one of the most nutritious food groups. It is recommended that you eat at least four to five servings of vegetables a day, in the form of sabzi, salad, soup, raita and juice. Soluble and insoluble fibre that is present in vegetables keeps our bowel movements regular. Red, orange and yellow vegetables have excellent antioxidant properties, and are valuable for people who want to lose weight. Beta-carotene and vitamins C and E in vegetables help inactivate free radicals and fight cancer.

Fruits

Fruits are expensive but their health benefits are now well-understood. You will find bananas in almost every Indian home, but greater importance is given to seasonal fruits. Fruits contain natural sugars, giving them a sweet taste. Like vegetables, fruits are high in fibre, vitamins and minerals. The intake of fruits needs to be monitored, though. Having the right fruit, at the right time, and in the right quantity is necessary to receive its maximum benefit.

Eating two to three fruits in a day is recommended. Try to avoid eating fruits with meals to ensure that there is no sudden rise of blood sugar leading to insulin resistance and storage of extra sugar as fat in the body. Diabetics should have fruits with high fibre nuts to stabilize their blood sugar and avoid sugar spikes.

The Secret to Eating Fruit

Eat fruits only on an empty stomach; never after a meal or even with bread. Eat fresh fruits and juices - avoid cans, packaged fruits or bottled concoctions. Drink fresh fruit juice, drink it slowly and let it mix with your saliva, before swallowing it. If we consume fruit the right way and in the right quantity first thing in the morning, it can help graying hair, balding and dark circles, boost energy levels and be great for our skin.

Milk and Milk Products

Rich in proteins, fats, carbohydrates and calcium, these form an important part of the Indian diet. Paneer, buttermilk and yoghurt made from toned milk, are healthy foods which are integral to the Indian diet. There are some desserts which can be prepared with milk, and if consumed only occasionally, should not hamper one's health.

Raita

You will find this dish in the cuisines of most parts of India. Raita is prepared by chopping or grating vegetables like cucumber, carrot, beetroot, radish, tomato, onion and mixing them with yoghurt. To this mix can be added chopped green chillies, and salt and sugar for flavour. The raita can be garnished with coriander before serving. It is used as a side-dish and provides an additional dash of fibre and proteins to the meal.

It is not just an accompaniment, and there is a reason why its served with Indian food. Like each spice has a job to do, so does raita. It is made with yoghurt, which provides protein and lines the stomach. A natural coolant, it helps digest food better, especially dishes like biryani that are difficult to digest.

Chutney

Dry or wet chutneys also serve as side-dishes in Indian cuisine along with roti-sabzi, or dal-rice, idli or dosa. A variety of chutneys are made from peanuts, flaxseeds, coriander, mint, sesame, kokum and coconut. A common method of preparing dry chutney is to roast the main ingredient and add spices to it as per your taste. For instance, sugar can be added for a sweet taste, tamarind or kokum to make it sour, and green or red chillies to make it hot. Grind the ingredients together and store them for eating later. Wet chutneys like coconut-coriander, tomato, tamarind, etc., are made fresh and consumed immediately.

Can Indian Food Benefit Our Health?

As I have mentioned earlier, the kitchen of every Indian family controls its health. Herbs and spices have a special place in the kitchen. Every Indian kitchen is equipped with a box with small compartments for spices that are used daily in cooking. These are mustard seeds, turmeric, red chilli powder, asafoetida, fenugreek seeds, kokum, tamarind and homemade garam masala.

The cures of several illnesses are in the hands of every Indian. You just need to know your foods well. Kick out the bad fats and carbohydrates, limit the sugars, and have the rest in balanced amounts—cereals, pulses, milk and milk products, nuts and oilseeds, fruits, vegetables, and non-vegetarian food too.

For common health complaints like cold and cough, sore throat, bloating, acidity, menstrual cramps and headaches, we actually don't need to run to a doctor. Indian spices contain powerful antioxidants which can provide relief from such complaints. Apart from spices, fruits and vegetables like guava, apple, orange, tomato, capsicum, amla, pineapple, papaya and so on are also excellent sources of antioxidants. If one decides to have proper portions of fruits and vegetables in one's regular diet, then one can develop a strong immune system to fight a range of illnesses.

As far as serious health issues are concerned, evidence shows that cardiovascular diseases, cancer, diabetes and high blood pressure are the leading causes of death in India. Indian foods, especially spices, have medicinal properties that can help cure several of these diseases.

Let's have a quick look at how spices, if consumed in correct proportions, can keep us away from illness.

Garlic

Healing compound: Allicin

Quantity to be consumed: Smash, cut or crush one to two cloves of garlic and have them daily.

How it helps:

- It lowers the risk of heart disease by 76 per cent by moderately reducing cholesterol levels and thinning the blood.
- It is an excellent source of antioxidants, which help fight cancer by flushing out carcinogens before they can damage cell DNA.
- It has anti-fungal and anti-bacterial properties which provide relief in the case of common cold, cough and fever.

Best ways to consume it: If you cannot eat it raw, add garlic to your soups, vegetables, salads, and vegetables juices.

Prevention is Better than Cure

'Indian food is medicinal and one of the most nutritious foods available when it comes to prevention and cure. Our family has used Indian food as a staple diet for years, and I strongly encourage people to make use of this amazing cuisine for their health and well-being.'
Vishal Gondal, CEO, GOQii

Turmeric

Healing compound: Curcumin

Quantity to be consumed: One teaspoon of turmeric powder or one curcumin tablet daily.

How it helps:

- It reduces inflammation caused by the growth of cancer cells and works like garlic in flushing out carcinogens, thereby stopping the growth of cancer cells.
- In studies on animals, curcumin has been shown to decrease the formation of beta-amyloid, which causes brain deposits characteristic in people with Alzheimer's disease.
- Being an amazing antioxidant, anti-bacterial and anti-fungal agent, it helps relieve infections that cause colds and coughs.

Best ways to consume it:

- Add half a tablespoon of turmeric to warm water and sip it. You can develop the habit of consuming turmeric in your children by adding it to their milk instead of the flavoured powders available in the market.
- You can also make tiny balls from a mixture of jaggery and turmeric. Cancer patients, however, are not allowed to consume sugar or jaggery.

Cinnamon

Healing compound: Polyphenols

Quantity to be consumed: Quarter to half a teaspoon of powdered cinnamon in a day.

How it helps:

- It is known to control blood sugar levels in people with diabetes.
- It burns body fat to some extent by increasing the metabolic rate.
- It helps in cutting down triglyceride and cholesterol levels, thus making it heart-friendly.
- Cinnamon is known to be packed with a high amount of antioxidants. Because of this, it helps reduce the proliferation of cancerous cells.

Best ways to consume it:

- Add one to two teaspoons of ground cinnamon to a hot cup of green tea and get double the dose of antioxidants.
- An inch of cinnamon can be added to your hot vegetable or lentil soup, stir-fried vegetables, curries, and in some rice preparations to add an exotic flavour.
- One teaspoon of cinnamon powder can be added to lukewarm lemon water and consumed early in the morning to help speed up your metabolism.

> ### Some Amazing Facts about Curry
>
> The earliest known mention of a curry—a spicy sauce with meat, vegetables and bread—is etched on tablets found in Babylon dating to around 1700 BC. Curries have been cooked for thousands of years, and an Indian curry may contain more health benefits than evident at first glance. Evidence suggests that it can benefit the heart, have a positive effect on people who have diabetes, and may even diminish cancer cells.

Indian Food and Cancer Cells

Cancer is a deadly disease characterized by the uncontrolled growth of abnormal cells. In the normal process of cell division, cells grow, divide to make new cells, and die. But in the case of cancer, abnormal cells keep growing and damaging other cells. Nutrients required to treat cancer are antioxidants like vitamins A, C and E, selenium and zinc to stop the proliferation of cancer cells, phytonutrients like lycopene and carotenoids to fight existing cancer cells, and fibre to form bulk and remove waster matter quickly so the carcinogen cannot act on it and aggravate the situation. Fibre also helps keep your blood sugar, cholesterol and blood pressure in control. Proteins are required for the growth and repair of cells.

It is widely accepted that in order to reduce the risk of cancer and combat it, we should incorporate a wide variety of fruits and vegetables in our diet. In Indian cuisine, vegetables are used widely, sometimes even as a meal in themselves.

Whole grains like oats, wheat, brown rice, barley and bulgar are excellent sources of good carbohydrates packed with high fibre.

Lentils and legumes like chickpea, black beans, peas and kidney beans are great sources of fibre and protein. They are also rich in folate and B vitamins. The role of folate in general is to repair damaged cells. This role signifies its importance in fighting dangerous cancer cells.

Nuts and seeds, like walnuts, almonds and flaxseeds, are rich sources of omega-3 fatty acids and phytosterols which helps the body fight cancerous cells.

The oleic acid in olive oil and the medium chain fatty acids in coconut oil help inactivate cancer cells.

The red-orange-yellow coloured fruits, especially berries, apples, papaya, and plums, are packed with antioxidants that help kill cancerous cells while leaving the healthy cells intact.

Broccoli, brussels sprouts, cauliflower and cabbage are cruciferous vegetables which contain an excellent set of antioxidants and polyphenols, such as hydroxycinnamic acid, kaempferol and quercetin, which fight cancer of the prostate and colon.

Almost all the spices in the Indian kitchen are packed with antioxidants. They have anti-inflammatory, anti-fungal and anti-bacterial properties which make them a necessity in the dietary checklist of cancer patients, especially curcumin.

On my stint in London for the TV show, 'Big Brother', I made friends with fellow contestant, Dirk Benedict, the American actor. He only ate brown rice and red kidney beans throughout his stay. When I quizzed him about it, he told me how he had cured himself of cancer just by eating that as his staple diet. He is alive today, and healthier than before.

When it comes to cancer, my approach is quite simple. Something in the body and its environment has changed, allowing cancer cells to grow and spread. It is important for the person to understand this and make changes so that the body's internal environment can change to one that is unfavourable for growth and spread of cancer cells. Cancer is the symptom of a sick body. Normally, one cell will multiply into two and then into four, so that there is exponential growth. But, at some point, it will shut off growth and just stay. Your liver grows to a certain size and remains that size. Your brain, your heart and all other cells grow to a certain size and stay that size. They have an inbuilt regulator that keeps the cells from growing more than a particular number. In the case of cancer cells, that regulator is turned off and so the cells just keep multiplying uncontrollably. Also, perhaps due to their physiological makeup, they absorb sugar in larger quantities than the normal cells. Cancer cells are basically rogue cells that are mutant, have damaged DNA and have escaped the guard, so to speak, of the immune system.

A cancer patient typically has to undergo chemotherapy and radiation, and they hope that this treatment will take care of their cancer and heal them. The problem lies here. Chemotherapy and radiation, as we all know, are so powerful and toxic that they affect the healthy cells in the body too, as well as its immunity. This is the reason why these treatments are likened to a double-edged sword. We are not against chemotherapy and radiation. They are required in many cases, but in many others, they may not be needed at all. If one opts for this line of treatment, the most important thing the the patient needs to do is help his or her body get through the harsh treatments by making lifestyle changes and introducing the right nutrition in their diet to change that body's internal environment. You have to do a lot more for yourself to help your body and not just rely on the treatments, which can eventually make you sicker.

Over the last few years, we have seen how Indian food and spices have shrunk tumours and arrested the growth and spread of cancer. We were amazed to hear from doctors that the Indian diet for their patients was working miracles. We continued to introduce simple Indian foods and spices to help the patients' bodies fight the cancer, though it is not just food and nutrition. Prevention and cure of cancer is also dependant on other lifestyle changes.

We are programmed from the day we are born to heal ourselves, provided we give our bodies the right nutrients and not poison ourselves with dangerous toxins. Most of the so-called success that doctors would claim in radiotherapy or chemotherapy treatments is based on shrinking a tumour. It does not address the underlying systemic problem. What you have in fact done is weakened the immune system's ability to deal with other cancers.

Chemotherapy also damages the brain. It causes 'chemo brain', which refers to thinking and memory problems as a result of chemotherapy. Every oncologist knows this to be the case. It also damages the kidneys and the liver. With chemotherapy, you are inflicting systemic damage on the body's ability to heal itself and remove toxins.

Like I said, we are not against chemotherapy, but if you choose to do this, ask your doctor all the questions you have to, get the answers, use logic, and support your treatment with solid nutrition and lifestyle changes.

Ten Things That Can Cause Cancer besides the Carcinogens Found in Food and Air

1. Obesity
2. Smoking
3. Internalizing stress or emotional distress
4. Lack of oxygen (incorrect and insufficient breathing)
5. Acidic bodies
6. Vaccinations
7. Heavy metals
8. Electromagnetic frequencies (EMF)
9. Poor nutrition, lack of physical activity and sleep
10. Anything that compromises immunity

Cinnamon Helps Diabetes and Cholesterol

Several studies have determined that consuming as little as half a teaspoon of cinnamon each day might reduce blood sugar, 'bad' cholesterol (low-density lipoprotein or LDL) and triglyceride levels by as much as 20 per cent in Type II diabetic patients who are not taking insulin.

Cinnamon, used extensively in the Indian diet, results in healthier blood. This amazing spice significantly reduces blood sugar levels in diabetics. Several studies have revealed that a diet high in spices like cinnamon, black pepper, and turmeric or curcumin, can do wonders for the heart and your overall health.

Cinnamon Can Sweeten Your Life without Causing Diabetes

'This spice with a peculiar taste has super anti-inflammatory power and has been shown to reduce arthritic pain. Not only that, it also helps curb the LDL and blood sugar levels drastically. Moreover, my personal experience shows that chewing a small piece of cinnamon helps cut down sweet cravings to a great extent. Cinnamon is a power spice! It has lots of hidden advantages to be explored.' Shimpli Patil, nutritionist and lifestyle coach

Prevention, Cure and Recovery from Diseases

Have you come across the terms 'acidic' and 'alkaline'? What these terms remind me of is my chemistry laboratory at school where we used litmus paper to check whether the given chemical was acidic or alkaline. Indian foods, too, are classified according to whether they are acidic or alkaline in nature.

The important thing to know is that we want to keep our bodies in an alkaline state at most times. Most diseases proliferate in an acidic environment, especially cancer. Joint problems and back pain occur more in an acidic body. Weight loss is slower in an acidic body. When the pH of your body becomes acidic, your body uses the calcium from your bones to neutralize the acidity. Basic chemistry will show that this leads to a deficiency of this vital mineral.

Let us go back to school for a bit. Do you remember the pH chart?

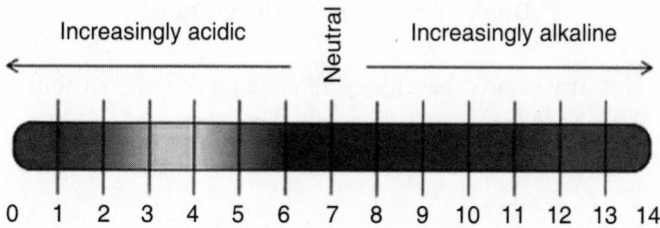

Alkalinity or acidity is measured by the pH value of body fluids. The pH scale extends from 0–14, 0 being most acidic and 14 being the most alkaline.

What we want to do for great health is to ensure our bodies stay alkaline. That's why the practice of squeezing a lemon over your food is a great one. Lemon is acidic in its raw state, but when it mixes with saliva, it becomes highly alkaline. The next time you suffer from acidity, have a glass of water with freshly squeezed lemon and you will feel better.

If you don't sprinkle lemon on your food, you can choose to drink a glass of lemon water after your meal, another great Indian habit. This will ensure efficient digestion and prevent bloating or gas formation.

Keep your body alkaline, and you stay in optimum health. This is one of the reasons why junk food and foods rich in salt and sugar can be bad for you. They are highly acidic in nature, besides being rich in the wrong kind of fats, chemicals and preservatives.

Want to lose weight faster? Keep your body alkaline.

Got a bad back or aching knees? Keep your body alkaline.

Don't Like Lemon or Allergic to It?

Here are some other highly alkaline foods that can shift your body from an acidic to alkaline state:

- Spinach
- Cucumber
- Bell peppers
- Broccoli
- Celery
- Avocado

End your meal with some salad sticks, and you will get your body's pH level in balance.

Acidic and Alkaline Foods

Extremely nutritious foods can be acidic. This does not mean we do not eat them. What it calls for is eating a balanced meal, which has alkaline-rich foods as well as acidic foods to bring about a perfect balance. The great Indian diet can bring about that balance.

The foods that are most alkaline are lemons, cucumber, papaya, melons, mangoes, grapes, fresh vegetable juices, garlic, onions, asparagus, broccoli and spinach.

Artificial sweeteners and sugars, refined white flour and sugars, chocolates, prunes, alcohol, aerated drinks, milk, cream, walnuts, peanuts and coffee are acidic in nature.

What you read as you go through the rest of the book will help you understand the benefits of Indian food and hopefully motivate you to adopt the great Indian diet.

Is the Great Indian Diet Only a Diet to Lose Weight?

The hype around diets over the last few years is probably one of the many reasons a lot of men, women and children drive themselves into depression. Worse than that, they lose their health in the process.

When it comes to your health goal, no matter what it is, your diet is a part of the larger jigsaw puzzle called 'lifestyle'.

What Does 'Diet' Mean?

The word 'diet' is associated with the feeling of developing eating habits that are time-bound and coupled with a strict food plan. But the actual meaning of diet is the food routine which a person follows daily. We believe in a lifestyle plan. It involves creating a food plan that revolves around your lifestyle, work, the quality of your sleep, the kind of exercise you do, your stress levels, your palate, and your personality. So much goes into designing the right food plan that works for your body, and most importantly, your mind.

Diet can be a depressing word, given the associations one forms with it. Difficult, deprived of one's favourite foods, where one consumes fewer carbohydrates and higher amounts of protein, feels hungry, battles cravings, and so on, are some of the common impressions one has of a 'diet' or a food plan. It need not be so. A food plan should be doable, make one happy, and fit easily into one's routine.

Origin of 'Diet'

The word 'diet' comes from the Middle English 'diete', from Latin 'diaeta' and from Greek 'diaita', which literally means the 'manner of living'.

Diet is your way of life and the choices you make to nourish and feed your body.

A good and healthy diet:

- Is easy to do and sustain
- Keeps you motivated
- Gives you nutrition
- Enables your body to absorb nutrition
- Fits into your lifestyle, no matter how hectic it is
- Works on the principles of moderation and compensation
- Helps you achieve and maintain a healthy weight
- Looks after the health of your hair and skin
- Prevents or cures diseases
- Builds strong immunity
- Keeps your vital organs and cellular system healthy

However, all our bodies are different and so is the diet suited to each one of us. Your diet will depend on various factors, such as:

- Where you live
- Your body type
- The kind of work you do
- How much you sleep
- How much physical activity you get
- Your stress levels
- Your mental and physical health
- Your good and bad habits

Now, does it make sense to Google a diet plan and blindly follow it?

Does it make sense to adopt the latest diet plan your friends are talking about?

Does it make sense to start randomly cutting out essential macronutrients such as carbohydrates, fats and proteins, because you believe that is the best way to lose weight?

All of us know people who rapidly lost weight and stunned their friends and families with fabulous bodies. We all get inspired to try and adopt what they did. We must respect those who lost weight the right way, by putting in effort and hard work, and being disciplined when it came to choosing between food that was good and bad for them. Not many of us might know that people might lose weight rapidly the wrong way, because all we talk about is the number of kilos they have shed. What is not shared are other aspects, like the amount of bone density lost in the process, the depletion of key vitamins and minerals (which will have severe consequences later in life) and the onset of depression caused by deprivation, extreme restriction, and the fact that the person knows that he or she will always have to work hard to keep the weight off.

Sounds pretty depressing, doesn't it? Over the years, we have seen clients and friends who started with a simple weight loss goal and ended up messing their lives so much that they needed sleeping pills and a whole array of other medication to fix what they broke in the process. If there's anything that will guarantee successful results, is discipline. That I assure you.

There is no short-cut when it comes to your health. The best and most expensive health clinics, foods, gyms and supplements cannot guarantee anything when it comes to fixing your health problems or in helping you achieve your health goals.

It all lies in your lifestyle and the choices you make. If there is ever a pill that claims to pull off the weight loss trick, that is the pill you should avoid. The simple thing that you need to remind yourself is: if it really worked, there would be no fat people in this world.

Yes, there are many great herbs, plants and spices that aid in healthy and quick fat loss, but all these work in conjunction with appropriate amounts of sleep and physical activity, as well as a strong and healthy mind. In *The Great Indian Diet*, we will discuss several of these fat-burning spices, herbs and foods.

Why Do We Have Diseases in India?

If the great Indian diet is as healthy as I am making it out to be, why then is there an alarming increase in the number of cancer, diabetes, cardiovascular and other diseases in India over the last few years?

Why are Indians living longer but suffering more?

Why are almost all diseases that have inflicted India related to poor diet and lifestyle?

Why are Indians earning more and also spending more on healthcare?

Why is the country getting more obese?

Why do non-meat eaters have extremely high sugar levels and cholesterol too?

Why is cancer rampant in urban areas?

Why is there an alarming increase in the number of obese children and children with diabetes, some as shockingly young as fourteen?

Why are there more gyms and more unhealthy people?

Why do we have more nutritionists and more confused people?

India is the country where yoga originated. Why, then, do we have increasing numbers of people with depression and other mind-related issues in the country?

Could the Indian diet be the cause of all of this?

We can write an entire chapter on what has changed in the last few years that has led to the above situation. In a nutshell, here is what has happened and is still happening.

A lot has changed and continues to change, in terms of lifestyle. We all know that change is inevitable, but then, there is good change and bad change.

Here is how Dr David L. Katz, Director of Yale University Prevention Research Center, explains it, 'As for the traditional Indian diet, I love it. For starters, it is all about nutritious food, mostly plants—just what we should all be eating. Fascinating medicinal properties have been ascribed to many native Indian spices, and science is confirming most such claims. as Indians have *abandoned* their native diet for a more Western diet, they have started succumbing en masse to obesity, diabetes and other chronic diseases. India should go back to embracing the culinary delight and health benefits of one of the world's great traditional cuisines.'

That's what happened and is happening. Our lifestyles have changed.

We began to use white refined sugar instead of the traditional and highly medicinal gur (jaggery).

We embraced the cleverly marketed olive oil and did away with super-nutritious local oils like rice bran, groundnut, mustard seed and coconut oils.

Margarine and butter replaced the extremely medicinal desi ghee.

We started adding more cream and oils to traditional recipes to make them 'richer' and taste better.

Whole grains like wheat, barley and millets were replaced with highly refined white flour to make Indian breads and snacks.

Rich desserts made with jaggery and nutritious dry fruits were replaced by and transformed into 'sugar-coated' or 'chocolate-covered delights'.

We moved from sea or rock salt to the highly refined table salt.

We began to feed our animals GM foods and inject them with hormones and antibiotics to increase their size and for mass production.

To grow crops faster, the amount of fertilizers used on them increased.

The import gates opened, flooding our markets with the very foods that Western nations were trying to get rid of.

Fast food joints sprung up all over the country, destroying the health of people nationwide.

The TV and video game culture hit us hard, robbing millions of people of valuable time that could have been saved and used to exercise, build relationships, sleep properly and just relax and enjoy the finer and more important things in life.

People who grew up on Indian foods have now transitioned to foods like pastas, noodles, pizzas, etc. There is nothing wrong with these foods when eaten once in a while and in moderation, but they should not replace the Indian diet, as they cannot provide the same kind of balanced nutrition that Indian food can.

As lives got busier, the need for quick fixes increased. Instead of resting out a headache, people began to indiscriminately pop pills, leading to the widespread abuse of medicines like painkillers, antacids, antibiotics and other pharmaceutical products.

The whey protein and supplement market boomed, cleverly, and in many cases falsely, 'educating' people about their uses and benefits. The increase in the numbers of kidney- and liver-related diseases could be related to the incorrect use of such products.

Change is Good, but at What Cost?

Some things listed above are not controllable, and the ever-increasing pollution levels in India do not help either. To manage our weight, cure and prevent diseases, feel and look good, and over and above just exercise and sleep well, we need to adopt healthy and balanced nutrition.

The great Indian diet can provide just that.

Before we begin to explore the Indian diet in detail, I think it is important for us to understand how food and lifestyle affect our weight and health.

It is important to know how we get fat, how we can burn fat, how we can boost our immunity, and how we can prevent and cure diseases in the simplest manner possible.

Part Two
What Is Going Wrong?

The Evils of the Food Industry

Every time you go to the store, you probably shop for the best foods available at the lowest prices. You might also take into account the time involved in cooking your meals. You might be a working person and living a busy life. If you are, you may feel that you do not have the time to cook, and as a result, you end up buying ready-made food and other packaged items. This may appear to be very convenient—just throw it in the microwave or open the package, and you have a ready-to-eat meal. But is this healthy? Not from a nutritional point of view. Unfortunately, this is how the food industry works.

When you go to a store, most of what you see on the shelves are processed foods. Food manufacturers include artificial ingredients in their products to not only increase their shelf life, but also to get you addicted to their products so that you keep returning to buy more—because the more you buy, the more money they make. What you do not realize about these products is that nearly all of them are made with ingredients that are bad for your health. They are loaded with preservatives, artificial ingredients, and chemicals that can cause cancer, heart disease and other ailments. Once you understand what such foods contain and what those chemicals do inside your body, you will appreciate knowing how to eat right, for yourself and for your family. If you take the time to read the list of ingredients on packaged foods carefully, you will discover that many of these are complex compounds, which are mostly chemicals that have been added to the food items.

The food industry corrupts our health for its own profits. You must realize that the industry is poised to make money. Maximum profit is what matters to manufacturers. There are facilities where food products are made in huge vats. The faster and cheaper they make the products, the sooner they can get into stores. And the sooner they can hit the shelves, the faster they will be bought and the more profits the manufacturers will make.

I remember making a trip to a food factory once. When I saw how the food was being made to be sold in stores, I realized why people get sick and even die from eating junk food. It was not until years later that I learnt that most food manufacturers create their products in exactly the same way. So, in a nutshell, when you buy ready-made food items in the store, all you are getting is a ton of artificial, man-made junk with little or no nutritional value. **The important lesson to learn is that if you must buy something ready-made, please read the label on the pack. The art of choosing what to buy is that the label should have fewer ingredients and natural preservatives.** The longer the list, the more you are complicating your health.

Oestrogenic Compounds

If you are having trouble getting rid of your belly fat, we have news for you. There are certain compounds called 'oestrogenic compounds' that cause your body to store excess fat. These compounds have been proven to be dangerous for both men and women. In women, they can affect the balance of the hormones oestrogen and progesterone, which in turn causes metabolic issues. The result is excess belly fat. In men, having excess oestrogenic compounds can lead to the accumulation of stomach fat that just will not go away. It can also lead to cancer and other diseases.

What causes this overload of oestrogenic compounds? Believe it or not, the culprit is soya. The food industry actively promotes soya as a health food, saying how much healthier your body would be if you consumed it regularly.

This is an outright lie. Soya is not, and never was, a health food. Do not let the food industry fool you. The people who claim that soya is good for you are those who make soya products. Soya contains some of the highest levels of pesticides among agricultural products. It is also a high source of phytoestrogens. If you consume a lot of soya, you will quickly find yourself suffering from hormonal imbalances.

Why We Eat the Wrong Foods

There are several reasons why we eat the wrong foods. Most people will claim right away that they do so when they are hungry. However, it is not so simple.

The habit of eating the wrong kinds of foods develops over a period of time. One of the reasons could be the easy availability of packaged foods. Available in every shop, it is convenient and cheap. Instead of looking for healthy food to eat, which might take time to prepare, we seek quick meals. We may want to satisfy our cravings instantly, so we stop at a McDonald's to grab a value meal. People often eat just because they get addicted to certain foods. The problem is that it often turns out to be overly processed and loaded with refined sugars. These are not good choices because such foods make your body release insulin and go into fat-storing mode.

At times, we also make the wrong choice by eating in order to deal with our emotions. Emotion does play a big part in making us eat the wrong foods. When we are low, we rush towards sugary or junk foods, thinking they will help us feel better. Can food make our everyday problems disappear? Of course not. This kind of escapism results in nothing but bad health.

Some people eat because they socialize, and the most common requirement while socializing is for people to share a meal. The problem is that when the meal is chosen, no one stops to think about the kinds of foods to buy or order. Invariably, people tend to consume foods with high sugar and oil content, not realizing that the body will end up storing these as fat. This is why many people struggle with obesity and health problems early in life. There is a way these patterns of behaviour can be prevented. It starts with altering your eating patterns. That is the first step, but as for the body, you can reverse what you have been doing to it by simply cleaning out your system and ridding it of the effects of years of food abuse.

How can you do this? By starting with a colon cleanse. Later in this book, I will share with you a simple detoxification plan compiled using Indian foods and spices. Use this plan to get a head start with your weight and health goals. The great Indian diet consists of some of the world's best foods, spices and herbs that can cleanse the body effectively.

Colon Cleanse and Detox

When you do a colon cleanse, you are in fact flushing out stored-up waste from the colon. It is important to have a clean colon. For one thing, having a clean colon will reduce your fat intake and thereby reduce your weight. Your energy levels will also increase.

By cleaning out the colon, you will eliminate waste such as fatty tissue, toxins, mucus and hardened fecal matter from your system. Whenever you do a colon cleanse, make sure you eat more fibre. Stay away from red meat and other non-fibrous foods. Do not eat out and avoid all salty and processed foods.

Now, let us look at how to detox your body. If you are not familiar with it, it is a way to clear your system of impurities, waste and toxins to keep you healthy. Any pollution, both indoor pollutants and outdoor toxins, and build-up matter, are removed from your body. Detoxing can be done by drinking juices. By doing so, you are not adding to the spread of toxins in your body while nourishing your body. When you research fruits and vegetables for detoxification, you will find there are many that can be used. Green vegetables, in particular, contain chlorophyll, which has a cleansing and healing effect on the digestive tract and the liver.

Foods That Are Bad for Health

I have spoken about what is wrong with the food industry and how we get tricked and addicted to foods that do our bodies no good. But what are these foods, and how do they affect our health?

Aerated Drinks

Sodas are full of sugar, unless they are of the diet variety, in which case they are full of artificial sweeteners. They also contain caffeine, and artificial colours and flavours. What really makes them bad for our health is that they have no nutritional value. The reason people drink them is because they like the taste. When considering soda, think about what it contains. Here is a breakdown of its ingredients:

- Carbonated water: This is plain water infused with carbon dioxide.
- Caramel colour: It is chemical, methylimidazole, and not natural.
- Natural flavours: These are mainly citrus flavours used for taste.

- Caffeine: For those who drink coffee, you know what this drug can do. It is a diuretic and stimulant that can be addictive.
- Phosphoric acid: When this is added to soda, it gives the liquid a tangy or sour taste by breaking down starch to sugar.
- High-fructose corn syrup: It is very unhealthy because it has no nutritional value. Instead, it has lots of calories. Those who consume it end up with heart disease as it causes the hardening of arteries. We will discuss this in detail later.

By drinking soda, you are loading up on sugar and calories. This is certainly not good if you want to lose weight. When you drink one can of soda, your pancreas produces and releases more insulin. This action takes the sugar out of your bloodstream and places it in your cells for energy. What happens next is that your insulin level rises. If nothing is done to alter this, your immune system weakens, eventually causing diabetes. This does not happen at once but over a period of time. It is something you need to be aware of.

When sugar is dumped into your cells, it gets stored as fat. And when more and more sugar is stored in these cells, it eventually results in weight gain.

Another reason soda is bad when consumed in excess is because of caffeine. Caffeine is a diuretic and will dehydrate you if you are not careful. It causes your kidneys to work harder to push the extra liquid out of your body. Caffeine also reduces the calcium in your body and increases your stress levels. It causes insomnia and nervousness.

It would be better if you reach for a glass of water, fruit juice, or even better, green tea, the next time you are thirsty.

Refined Sugar

Refined sugar constitutes all those sugars that have been processed. Processing refers to when a substance goes through a purification process during which its impurities and coarseness are removed. Refining separates the sugar (sucrose) from plant materials, which is followed by the removal of unwanted materials from the sugar.

During the processing of sugar, washing, boiling, centrifuging, filtering and drying are carried out. At the end of this process, all nutritional elements are gone from the sugar. What remains is 95 per cent sucrose and insignificant materials that have no nutritional value. What is even worse is that this mixture goes through another refinement wherein it is bleached with lime and carbon dioxide. After this process is completed, the material is whitened. What emerges a the end of all the processing and refining is table sugar, or a sweet substance with no nutritional value. It is simply junk food.

Refined sugar has no nutritional value and only tastes good. It is the most prevalent reason for weight gain, especially in women. One reason why refined sugar is consumed so much is because it is addictive. The minute you stop eating refined sugar, you will notice your body weight go down. You will even feel better.

Artificial Sweeteners

Artificial sweetener is exactly what the name suggests. It is made of chemicals that taste like sugar. Various artificial sweeteners are available in stores. Their ingredients include sorbitol, saccharin, aspartame and sucrolose. You should know that artificial sweeteners cause weight gain by disrupting your body's natural hormones. They mess with the brain, fooling it into thinking that the body is about to consume a heavy load of calories. So, the brain gets activated and works up the metabolism. Unfortunately, the calories never come, but the body stays revved up only for a short time. In the meantime, the chemicals in the artificial sweeteners begin to accumulate in the body and cause it to store fat, as well as inflicting damage to certain cells.

Artificial sweeteners have also been known to cause the following conditions:

- Cancer
- Brain tumours
- Kidney and liver damage

Processed Foods

If we buy foods that have already been cooked and treated with chemicals, we are feeding our bodies nothing but junk. This stresses the body and results in the development of diseases like diabetes, heart disease and other illnesses. It really does not take much to understand what processed foods can and will do to you if you consume them in large quantities. By doing so, you will, in fact, be killing yourself slowly. If you find yourself in the situation where you constantly buy processed and refined foods, take a break. Force yourself to stop buying them. Instead, go to the vegetable and fruit aisle of the supermarket, and stock up on fresh vegetables and fruits. By doing this, you will notice just how much healthier you will become, not to mention the unwanted pounds that will melt away quickly too.

As Dr Gloria Gilbere, a 'wholistic rejuvenist' says in her book, *When Food Becomes Your Enemy*, 'When food we eat is devoid of enzymes through cooking or processing, digestion is compromised, and the food becomes toxic as it ferments and decomposes—settling too long within our body and eventually being absorbed as toxic composite. Lack of good digestion stresses the liver and immune system, causing the breakdown of overall immune defenses, which later manifests as serious disorders. Cooking and heating destroys all enzymes—as does food processing—accounting for the increased rate of digestive disorders. If food is processed, it has been heated. This processing does not take into account the food additives and preservatives that also may break down enzymatic activity.'

Evil Sugar

Sugar is the devil; I mean refined sugar. Sucrose is also included in this. Any type of sugar is dangerous to your health because it can cause many illnesses and diseases in your body, including cancer, diabetes and excessive weight gain. There are many types of sugars to avoid. I covered these sugars extensively in a previous section, so

I will not go over them here. What I would like to talk about is a special type of sugar that I have only briefly mentioned earlier.

It has been called 'killer sugar' by many nutritionists. I guess you are wondering what it is exactly. What I am referring to is a sugar found in more food products than you realize. These include sodas, breakfast syrups, fruit juices, ketchup, sweetened cereals, cakes, cookies, pasta sources, and so much more.

The evil sugar I am talking about is corn syrup with a high content of fructose. Here are the facts. High-fructose corn syrup is a commonly used sweetener today due to its low cost. What makes it extremely harmful is the way the body metabolizes it. It is not processed in our bodies the way other sugars are. This sugar gets stored as fat. Your body cannot consume it because it really cannot determine its chemical breakdown. So, the sugar simply does not get digested.

The content of high-fructose corn syrup turns into fat and soon gets circulated throughout the blood stream. Before long, its contents begin sticking to the walls of veins and arteries. After a while, the blood vessels get clogged, preventing blood from reaching the heart, and eventually causing a heart attack.

If you want to eat something sweet, buy products that use raw honey, molasses or organic maple syrup. The sweetener that is healthy for you and will not cause weight gain is Stevia. Why is it so? It is a natural, non-caloric herb that has been used for thousands of years in South America. People there dry the herb and powder it. When you taste it, you realize how sweet it is. Those who have tried Stevia claim it is much sweeter than sugar. And there are no known side-effects of it. So, instead of using artificial sweeteners that can kill you, use a herb that has been known to be good and is completely natural.

Are You a Sugar Addict?

Many people are sugar addicts. What exactly is the definition of a sugar addict? Primarily, it is someone who loves to eat anything sweet. If you are a sugar addict, you better take heed of what I am saying here, for it may save your life.

You may not know this, but much of the food you see on the shelves today contains refined sugars and other overly processed ingredients. Most people eat as much as 63 kilos of sugar a year and get another 18 per cent of their calories from consuming white flour. Is it any wonder the obesity rate is higher than it has ever been before? What most people do not realize is that the fix they get from sugar only lasts a few hours. Then it causes you to crash. The results are devastating for your body. Sugar addiction is like any other form of addiction. For the sake of your body, you have to go through a withdrawal process to get over your sugar addiction. Since it is part of your lifestyle and habit, you need to work hard to overcome it. You could take the help of experts to understand its underlying causes and hopefully make the decision to fight it.

If you can treat the causes of your addiction, you will be able to cope with it much better. You will be surprised at how great you feel when you give up sugar. The main reason why sugar is addictive is because of its inherent sweetness. It also gives you an initial high, which wears out in a little while, resulting in a crash. Then, you need to consume more sugar to get that high again, and so the cycle continues.

The truth is that you really do not get energy from sugar. What you feel most of the time is the effect of high blood sugar. This is a false notion of feeling energetic. All you end up feeling is exhausted, anxious and moody. If you give up your sugar addiction, you can lower your risk of diabetes, hypertension, stroke and heart attacks. Subsequently, your metabolism will also become stable and boost normally, thereby burning all the fat and sugar in the body. The result is loss of body weight. If you are serious about losing weight and feeling great, you owe it to yourself to stop consuming sugar. To help you do this, here is a plan:

1. Start your day with a protein, fat and phytonutrients. Phytonutrients, also called phytochemicals, are natural bioactive compounds found mainly in fruits and vegetables. Maybe you could grab an apple or carrot, or have a bowl of berries with protein and fat. Do not forget to drink plenty of water throughout the day.

2. Eat three meals a day, along with two snacks. Make sure the snacks consist of nuts, seeds, vegetables or fruit. Do everything you can to stay away from sugary substances.

3. Make it a point to include L-Glutamine in your diet. L-Glutamine is an amino acid. It is used in the body to synthesize protein, regulate the acid–base balance of the kidney, provide cellular energy, among other things. You will find L-Glutamine

     in foods such as beef, chicken, eggs, cabbage, beetroots, beans, spinach, parsley and miso.

4. Each time you think about sweets, distract yourself by taking a walk or talking to someone. Keep your mind active for about ten to twenty minutes. This is usually how long the cravings last.

5. Eat a piece of fruit. This is the best way to avoid sugar. Fruit contains natural sugar that is healthy for you.

6. Drink tulsi tea with jaggery, ginger tea or even green tea with lemon, honey and jaggery.

7. When you go to the store, have someone with you so that when you reach for sugary products, the person stops you. Better yet, have someone else shop for you. This way, you will be certain of not bringing sugary products into the house.

8. Talk to people about your addiction. Join a support group. Do not try to deal with it alone. Deal with your emotional issues with sugar by getting help from someone else, especially someone who has also overcome the addiction.

If you take these steps, you will find your addiction to sugar gradually disappearing, and you will not crave it any more. Many people have done this and been successful.

The Truth about Milk

Another topic that seems to get a lot of attention is milk and milk fat. We all drank milk as babies and continue to do so in adulthood. You probably drank milk in school, in the morning with cereal, and in your favourite shake. You may do so even now. So what is wrong with drinking milk?

Here is the scoop. On one hand, there are cows that are fed growth hormones in order to increase their milk production. They are also fed antibiotics to decrease their risk of infections. These hormones and antibiotics end up in the milk they produce and which we eventually drink, thereby allowing them into our bodies. This is one of the main reasons why young girls put on weight rapidly and reach puberty earlier than they are supposed to.

There are also cows that are grass-fed, but the milk that is taken from them is put through a process of pasteurization and homogenization. In this, the milk is heated to high temperatures, and the good fat is broken up, and in some cases, removed, leaving the bad fat behind.

A Milk Substitute

I would suggest omitting milk and milk products if you are prone to coughs and colds, as it increases mucous formation.

But that is my personal opinion. Ayurveda suggests hot milk and turmeric for colds and coughs, but I have substituted it with ginger, lemon, black pepper, sea salt and honey with a quarter teaspoon of turmeric. It is a great antidote for coughs and colds, and tastes great too.

The best way around this would be to use non-fat milk, organic milk, raw milk or other kinds of milk, like almond milk. Almond milk is great because it has vitamins and minerals, along with calcium. When you go to the store to purchase milk, read the label carefully. Avoid any product that has high fat content, preservatives or any other additives. It could affect your health and your weight.

I hope this helps you understand how to drink milk and what kind of milk to opt for. This is also important for understanding the concept of fat, weight loss and your body. In a country like India, where milk is integral to our daily diet, it is important to know the kind of milk that is available to us now. Understand the pros and cons, and make an informed choice.

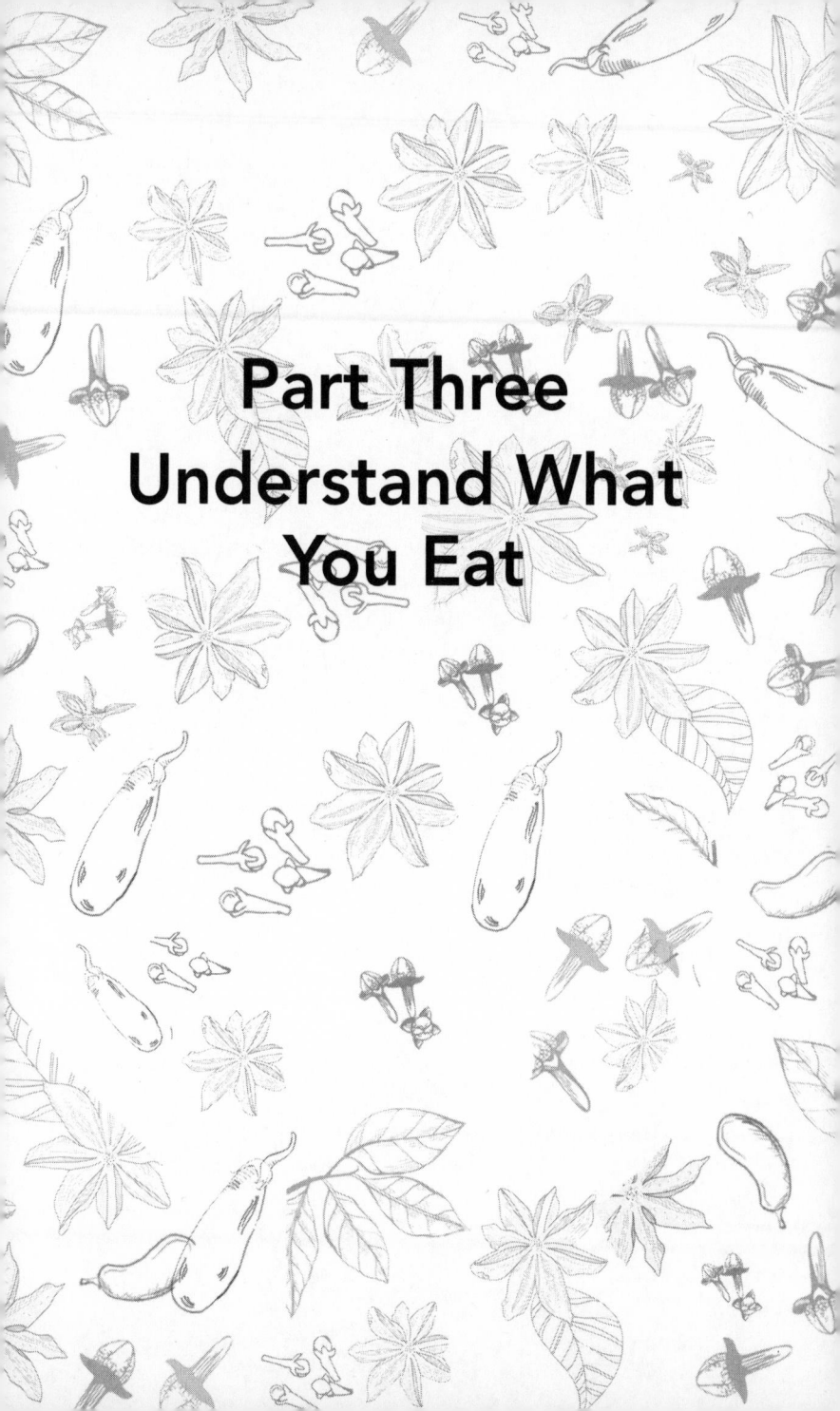

Part Three
Understand What
You Eat

The Components of a Healthy Meal

You may think it doesn't matter what you eat. Well, it does. If you eat anything you want, it will show on your body. If you eat the right foods, you will start losing weight until you fit into those jeans you've been hiding in your closet. Take the example of the Eskimos. They consume a lot of high-fat foods, including whale blubber, seal fat, cold water fish and organic meats. Yet, they don't suffer from heart ailments or any other diseases, and are certainly not obese. Have you thought why? One of the reasons for this is because the foods they eat are natural and not processed. Also, consider the Pacific Islanders. They are known to consume coconut fat, which is 90 per cent saturated fat. They do not have any diseases, simply because they don't touch foods that are processed. People in different countries eat differently. Each country consumes a certain level of fats, proteins and carbohydrates. However, what is common is that there originally wasn't a culture of eating refined or processed foods in the history of any country. None of us were created to eat refined and processed foods. Our bodies thrive best on local, fresh and organic foods.

If you take a closer look at the medical history of India, you will find that heart disease, stroke, diabetes and many other diseases were not rampant until refined and processed foods began to be consumed in large quantities. In other words, when food manufacturers began to deliver refined flour, refined sugar and refined or hydrogenated vegetable oils, is when people started getting such diseases, or at least these diseases became more common than before.

Now you know why the food that we eat matters. In fact, your life and body size depend on it. So, keep in mind that you are what you eat and you'll find out how your body responds to the foods you feed it. Let's talk about the various components of our diet and how they affect our health.

Carbohydrates

If you are avoiding carbohydrates because you think doing so is an easy way to lose fat, you are wrong. By not having carbohydrates, you are depriving yourself of a key and vital element of nutrition. Fat loss is never about extreme restriction. People cut down on carbohydrates but make no attempt to cut down on sugary foods and treats. Sometimes, eating fewer carbs at night, especially if you cannot keep a long gap between dinner and bedtime, is a good idea as your body needs more protein and fats at night to carry on its bodily functions while you are asleep. Of course, there are good and bad carbs. Good carbs are required for your health and fat loss, and bad carbs can damage your health and immunity and make you put on weight.

The great Indian diet includes some of the most nutritious carbohydrates known to man. To maintain a fast metabolism, we need a balanced diet that comprises all the macronutrients—carbohydrates, proteins and good fats. The absence of good carbs can cause sleep disorders and behavioural changes, along with low energy and fatigue. These symptoms can be mistaken for low food intake, making people consume more calories.

Some amazingly healthy Indian carbs are:

1. Brown and Red Rice

Unmilled, unpolished brown rice is extremely nutritious. It is a great source of selenium, magnesium, manganese and tryptohpan (a natural sleep inducer, the reason you may feel drowsy after eating rice). Wheat contains more protein than rice, but the quality of rice protein is better. Rice is the most easily digestible food, yet many people blame it for their weight gain. The process of polishing brown rice to make it white, and therefore attractive, destroys almost 70 per cent of all its B vitamins, chromium, zinc, fibre and essential fatty acids. Whole brown rice is, in fact, excellent for maintaining lower cholesterol levels. Selenium in brown rice is known to possibly prevent cancer. Rice is also rich in magnesium, which reduces the severity of asthma and migraines; it lowers blood pressure, calms the nerves and reduces the risk of heart disease and stroke. Rice is free of allergy-causing gluten, which is present in wheat.

2. Amaranth

Amaranth, also called chaulai, is the least allergenic of all grains. Even though it is one of the most nutritious grains on this planet, it is almost a forgotten food, except in India.

High in protein, it contains amino acids not found in other grains. It is also termed a 'brain food' as it is rich in fibre and minerals like calcium, iron, magnesium, potassium, zinc, copper and manganese. It also contains vitamins A, C, E, B_2, B_6, and folic acid.

Amaranth has more iron and calcium than wheat and milk, respectively. It contains a form of vitamin E that can lower cholesterol. An important thing to note is that people who suffer from kidney disease, arthritis, gout and stones should go easy on this grain as it contains oxalic acid.

3. Wheat

Apart from being rich in fibre and tryptophan, wheat is a great source of manganese, magnesium and potassium. Potassium plays a key role in maintaining optimum blood pressure. Wheat bran is a bulk laxative, and helps with regular bowel movements. Whole wheat is rich in high-quality vitamin E, which is essential for healthy skin and hair.

Whole wheat is also a true anti-cancer food. Among all the grains, only wheat bran counters colon cancer by adding bacteria enzymes in the stools.

Wheat also contains gluten, which some people are allergic to or simply lack the ability to digest. Gluten is found in many other grains too, like oats, barley and rye.

Some people say they are gluten-intolerant, but this needs to be tested correctly. In some cases, the health of their digestive systems might have been affected due to poor nutrition and lifestyle, making their systems too weak to digest not just gluten but many other foods as well. If you begin the process of making your digestive system healthier, you may find that you can freely consume wheat.

Wheat must be aged before consumption. That is how people had it up to seventy years ago. Aged wheat is easier for the body to break down. The ageing time has decreased and packaged wheat is being bought off the shelf. This is one of the main reasons for gluten intolerance.

Interestingly, women who eat more wheat have their oestrogen levels in control. This is important because an excess of oestrogen can give rise to fibroids, breast cancer and dangerous cysts. Wheat contains lignans, as do brown rice and oats. They maintain a friendly and healthy environment in the intestines and protect against many degenerative diseases, including cancer.

4. Barley

Barley is an extremely healthy grain and a great source of fibre and selenium. It lowers cholesterol and triglyceride levels in our blood. Due to its high fibre content, barley has a low glycemic index and is recommended for people with diabetes. This grain can keep you feeling full for a long time, making it a great weight loss food. Barley consumption is known to prevent gall stones and maintain the health of the liver. Its selenium content is good for the health of the prostate and the silica in it strengthens bones. Barley is also an excellent grain for pregnant women.

To flush out excess water that the body might retain, boil some barley in water, add some fresh lemon to it, and drink the concoction. It helps alleviate the symptoms of premenstrual syndrome (PMS) and can even be consumed after your menstrual cycle. Boiled barley can be eaten with dal or lentils, cooked with mixed vegetables, or added to soup to make a nutritious meal.

5. Corn

Corn contains folic acid, which helps lower homocysteine that causes damage to the arteries. A diet rich in fibre and folate is linked to reduced chances of colon cancer. Corn is a rich source of vitamins B_1, B_5 and C, as well as phosphorous and manganese.

6. Millets

Rich in fibre, protein, manganese and magnesium, this grain can keep you full for a long time and decrease your total intake of calories. During digeston, it breaks down and releases energy that can keep you feeling strong and energetic throughout the day.

7. Oats

Oats are an excellent weight loss and heart-friendly food. These are rich in selenium, manganese, fibre, vitamins and protein. Oats contain 'beta glucan', which can lower cholesterol levels rapidly. Consuming oats regularly is great for enhancing immunity. Rich in antioxidants, it keeps the heart and arteries healthy. Beta glucan also lowers and regulates blood sugar levels, making it a great food for diabetics. The soluble fibre present in oats improves digestion and prevents constipation, piles, colon cancer and gastrointestinal disorders, and also helps remedy these disorders. Consumption of oats is also a possible solution for insomnia, due to the presence of tryptophan and magnesium in them.

Proteins

How much protein do we really need? Is it true that the Indian diet cannot provide sufficient protein to the human body? Certain Indian foods, when used in combination with others, provide all the protein required by the body.

I see a lot of people on high protein diets gulping up to three protein shakes a day, and they are not even body-builders. A lot of people consume more protein than what their bodies require. Anything in excess is bad for your health. Excess protein that does not get utilized by the body is converted to fat. It also puts a load on your kidneys. What does this mean? The human body is capable of absorbing only a certain amount of protein at a time. So, forget about all those whey proteins that boast of more than 20 or 30 grams of protein per scoop. **Most bodies can absorb only around 15 to 17 grams of protein at a time**. What happens to the excess protein? It goes waste. However, if you are using good-quality whey for convenience's sake, that's a different story. I have parents coming up to me and asking me to select a whey protein for their kids because they feel sleepy at school or are not growing. That is not the solution.

The human body needs 0.8–1 gram of protein per kilo of your body weight. If you weigh 60 kilos, you need 60 grams of protein in a day. Such quantities can easily be obtained from a balanced Indian diet. Of course, if you are a body builder or an athlete, this amount per kilo of your body weight would be higher, but that's a different story. In those cases, you follow a specially designed sports nutrition plan, which has other supplements and foods to give you a balanced diet.

It is true that protein fills you up and keeps you from feeling hungry for a longer period of time, but that job is best left to the fibre in our food. Fibre is also responsible for cleaning and detoxifying your system without putting extra load on your kidneys.

If you think you'll become leaner by consuming more protein, there are other things to look at that contribute to a lean physique. The carbohydrates and fat ratios in your diet, the kind of exercise you do, the amount and quality of sleep you get, your stress levels and your mental health are far more instrumental in making you lean. Your body is the best indicator of your health and deficiencies, if any. You will know if you listen to it. The following are some of the signs your body may give you if you are deficient in protein:

- You are tired when you shouldn't be
- You feel weak when you exercise
- You are flabby when you should be toned or muscular
- You get injured quickly and take long to recover
- You have hair fall issues
- Your skin is not healthy

The reasons stated above can also be caused by various other deficiencies, but with regard to your body and protein, try and use these signs to determine if your protein intake is enough.

Lack of protein weakens the body and damages the nervous system, whereas excess protein produces toxins and acids and can damage the liver, kidney and digestive system. There are nine kinds of essential amino acids. A complete protein is one that comprises all nine. Eggs are an example of a complete protein food. Meat and fish are also complete proteins. Legumes and soybean are rich in good-quality protein. Amaranth is the highest quality plant-based protein that is also easily digestible. The combination of brown rice and rajma is a complete and high-quality protein food.

Plant foods individually do not contain all the nine essential amino acids, but combining them with other foods can provide high-quality protein that is sufficient to build a lean and healthy body and burn fat at the same time.

Dal and roti (legumes and wheat) or dal and chawal (legumes and brown rice) are great combinations that contain all nine amino acids required by your body. The following are some everyday foods that can boost your protein levels:

- Soybean
- Nuts (almonds, walnuts, peanuts and cashew nuts)
- Seeds (flax, sesame, sunflower and pumpkin)
- Green peas
- Spinach and green, leafy vegetables

- Milk and dairy products
- Whole grains (wheat, millets, bajra, ragi, amaranth and so on)
- Grams
- Beans
- Moong
- Alfalfa
- Mushrooms
- Dry fruits
- Yoghurt
- Paneer (Indian cottage cheese)
- Tofu
- Brown rice
- Dals (lentils)

These are whole foods, rich in protein and other vitamins and minerals, and which are found all across the Indian subcontinent.

Fats

I often see people devour large bowls of salad without dressings or oils. Have you ever thought of how these nutrients will be absorbed into the body?

We strongly believe that the recent fad of trying to lose weight by cutting out fats from the diet has to end. People who go on low-fat diets are destroying their health and losing weight in an unhealthy way. While talking to people who were on low-fat diets, we learnt that although they were losing weight, they were depressed, frustrated, irritable and unhappy with the way they were living. To top it all, they looked older and felt fatigued. Women who go on low-fat diets tend to suffer from hormonal complications.

My mother and grandmother would always encourage me to eat nuts and homemade ladoos, which made me get angry with them. Whenever I asked for extra papad or puri, or any fried stuff, they would tell me how oily food is harmful for health. I am sure you remember those days when you would ask for snacks in the evening, and your grandmother would open a big jar and give you a handful of dry fruits or peanuts or ghee and jaggery ladoos, instead of letting you go out and snack on chips and samosas. Ladoos, dry fruits, chips and samosas all contain fats. But there is one huge difference between these fats, which is why it is extremely important to learn about different kinds of fats. There are two types of fats—'good' fats and 'bad' fats.

Catch 'em young

I remember we had to ask Mom's permission before we had chips, wafers, chocolates and fried stuff. If she said 'no', it was no, till the age of ten. She inculcated discipline and that's paid off today.

Please negotiate and inculcate the right eating habits in your kids. You would rather play 'bad cop' now than be the reason for bad health later for your kids.

Start now. It's never too late. What you teach them forms habits, good or bad, and habits die hard.

Good fats are the essential fats which are required for healthy brain functioning, a strong immune system, and to maintain the body's hormonal balance and its energy production. Bad fats are those which clog our arteries and cause internal inflammation. All we need to do is, choose the right kind of fat and consume it in the right way.

Fats are broadly classified as:

1. Unsaturated fats (good fats)
2. Saturated fats (bad fats)
3. Trans fats (bad fats)

Unsaturated fats are further divided into polyunsaturated (omega-3 and omega-6) and monounsaturated fats. They help build cell membranes and form the exterior protective covering on each cell. They reduce LDL (bad cholesterol) more than they lower HDL (good cholesterol), thereby improving your cholesterol profile. What makes them even more beneficial is that they also lower triglycerides.

Sources of good fats are flaxseeds, walnuts, canola oil, and fatty fish like salmon, mackerel and sardines.

To distinguish one kind of fat from another, it is recommended that you develop the practice of reading labels before purchasing any product. If you come across terms like 'saturated fats' or 'trans fats', replace the product on the shelves. These are bad fats which harm our body in the following ways:

- They increase the acetate fragments in the body, which in turn leads to an increase in the production of cholesterol.

- They tend to clump together and form deposits in the body, along with protein and cholesterol, and get lodged in blood cells and organs leading to health problems like obesity, heart disease and cancers of the breast and colon.
- They build up in the arteries causing them to narrow, a condition that is called atherosclerosis and can consequently lead to major heart problems.
- Trans fat is made by adding hydrogen to vegetable oil through a process called hydrogenation, which makes the oil less likely to spoil but difficult to digest.
- These raise your bad (LDL) cholesterol and lower your good (HDL) cholesterol.

Sources of saturated fats include cheese, butter, cream, and red meat. Saturated fat is also found in tropical oils such as palm oil, coconut oil and cocoa butter.

After going through the above material, I am sure you too will stop quarrelling with your mother and grandmother about giving you ladoos made from ghee, dry fruits and nuts, which are all rich in the good fats.

Saturated Fat Is Wrongfully Accused

Let us not blame only saturated fats and trans fats for compromising your health by weight gain and clotting in the arteries. If you stop eating all fats, but continue to binge on junk foods made from refined wheat flour, cheese and sugar, like breads, pizzas, burgers, biscuits, cakes, pastries, and mithai, then you still run the risk of developing dreadful diseases. The reason is that all these products increase your blood sugar and thereby your insulin, leading to an increase of fat storage in your body.

The idea of avoiding all fats because they make you fat or clog your arteries is a nutritional myth. Everybody needs some amount of fat to stay healthy, lose weight and feel good. In addition to providing energy, there are some essential fats that function in our bodies as components for nerve cells in the brain and heart, and are important for producing hormones. They are also essential for transporting vitamins, minerals and hormones to each cell in the body.

There are, of course, good fats and bad fats that you should know about. Trans fats and hydrogenated fats are bad for your health, heart and weight. So are highly refined oils. Eating commercially made French fries is probably the worst food to feed yourself or your children. Then there are essential fatty acids (ESAs) found in vegetables, nuts, seeds and plants that are required for your health and can actually turn your body into a fat-burning machine. These fats are found in cooking oils used in Indian cooking. The sad part is that people today are moving towards oils used more commonly in Western countries and imported oils. Coconut oil and ghee have been pushed aside over the last few years, because it was claimed that they cause heart problems and obesity.

Olive oil is great for health but does not suit Indian cooking. In fact, it can do more damage to your health if it is heated to high temperatures while cooking Indian food.

Indians also force themselves to consume fish oil supplements, thinking that it is the only good source of omega-3 fatty acids. However, it is interesting to note that high-quality omega-3 fatty acids are found in the following:

- Flaxseeds or flaxseed oil
- Walnuts
- Pumpkin seeds
- Cloves
- Wheat germ
- Broccoli
- Green, leafy vegetables
- Spinach
- Eggs
- Fish
- Mustard oil

What you read next should hopefully convince you to actually include coconut oil and ghee in your diet. Traditional Indian cuisine extensively made use of these two good fats, and Ayurveda even prescribed these fats to heal and prevent disease.

Ghee

It comprises short, medium and long chain fatty acids, which means it contains both saturated and unsaturated fats. Ghee, when prepared from cow's milk, has the highest natural source of CLA (conjugated linoleic acid), which helps burn the stubborn fat in your body. Being rich in antioxidants such as vitamin A, D, E and K helps build up immunity, which is why it is given to newborns who are more susceptible to infections. Research shows that the consumption of ghee in limited amounts helps in cancer treatment due to the antioxidants in it. Butyric acid in ghee helps reduce inflammation, particularly in the gastrointestinal tract, aiding in proper digestion. It gives us healthy skin and eyes too, because of its high vitamin content.

However, we need to take care that we do not consume ghee in large quantities. It is better than oil and butter and can replace them whenever possible. I have recently started using ghee instead of butter while making sandwiches.

Shilpa's Recipe for Homemade Ghee

My mom used to collect malai (cream) that forms over milk and freeze it. When around a kilo had been collected, she would bring the cream to room temperature and churn it till the whey separated and turned to butter. If you don't want to go through the process of collecting cream, you can get readymade white butter from a local milk vendor.

Take the white butter and heat it on a low flame. Once you see the base of the vessel turning brown, add a pinch of salt (as per taste). After you see the ghee come to a boil, add a couple of tulsi (basil) leaves and two paan (betel nut) leaves for extra aroma and a golden colour. Let them fry, and you will see a brown tea-like decoction at the base of the vessel. Strain it, and your homemade ghee is ready. That's it. Pure organic ghee.

Keep in mind that these benefits are attached only to pure homemade ghee prepared without any preservatives or vegetable fats. Store-bought ghee or ghee that is prepared with artificial methods will not be in the same category as pure ghee.

Coconut Oil

Coconut oil is used extensively in tropical countries, especially India, Sri Lanka, Thailand, the Philippines and so on, which also produce it in vast quantities. At one time, coconut oil was also popular in Western countries like the US and Canada. However, in the Seventies, a propaganda campaign against coconut oil was begun by the corn oil and soya oil industries which maintained that coconut oil was harmful for the human body due to its high saturated fat content. It is only in the past decade that people have begun questioning the claims of this propaganda. Traditional Indian food uses coconut oil, especially the cuisine of South India.

Shilpa's Tips

I am a Mangalorean. So I've been brought up on coconut oil. Try the cold-pressed variety. It doesn't have the strong aroma of regular coconut oil.

Some qualities of coconut oil include:

- Aids in Weight Loss: Research shows that the medium chain fatty acids present in coconut oil go directly to the liver to get converted into energy, instead of circulating in the blood and settling in the body as fat. This means that the body does not get the chance of storing coconut oil as fat and gain weight, but instead it gives you an energy kick. It is also known to boost your metabolism and aid in burning more calories, which in turn keeps your weight in check.

- Bone Health: Coconut oil improves the body's ability to absorb minerals like calcium and magnesium, which are the prime components of our bones. Research shows that it reduces oxidative stress in the bone, ensuring there is no structural damage to the bones.

- Brain Booster: Research has shown that ketone bodies increase in patients with Alzheimer's disease and cognitive impairment improves with regular administration of coconut oil.

- Hair and Skin: Coconut oil has always been used as a skin moisturizer, especially during winter. In the early times, when there were no expensive creams and moisturizers in the market, people would apply coconut oil on dry skin to bring back its glow. The medium chain fatty acids present in coconut oil enable it to smoothen dry skin. Omega-3 fatty acids—capric, caprylic and lauric acid—have disinfectant and anti-microbial properties, making coconut oil a prime treatment for skin-related problems like psoriasis, dermatitis, eczema, among others.

- Diabetes Friendly: The medium chain fatty acids in coconut oil helps stabilize blood sugar levels by improving the secretion of insulin, thus promoting effective utilization of blood glucose.

- Improves Digestion: Medium chain fatty acids are quick and easy to break down during digestion. Coconut oil is found to give relief in digestive disorders like irritable bowel syndrome, ulcerative colitis, gastritis, diverticulosis and constipation. Coconut oil helps kill harmful bacteria, candida or parasites, and thereby cleans up the digestive system and makes it healthy.

- Stress Reduction: Many of us might have had this experience. When we return after a tiring day, our mother quickly opens the coconut oil bottle and begins massaging our head. It certainly keeps our stress under control and enables us to sleep soundly.

The Great Indian Diet Comprises Excellent Cooking Oils

Cooking oil is inevitable while preparing a dish. Whether it is salad or main course, you need to use oil. But choosing the right cooking oil can save you from heart disease, cholesterol blockage, obesity and digestive problems.

Cooking oil is either obtained from animals or vegetables. Vegetable oil is hands down a healthier eating option. There are several vegetable-based cooking oils in the Indian market. Below, we have explained the benefits of each oil and how it should be used.

1. Rice Bran Oil

Rice bran oil is extracted from the hard outer layer of rice. It has a high smoking point, is yellow in colour and is used to stir fry as well as deep fry. Rice bran oil is rich in monounsaturated and polyunsaturated fats and is free of trans fats, which is a ratio very close to the recommendations made by the American Heart Association for Indians. Rice bran has an antioxidant named oryzanol, which makes it effective in stabilizing cholesterol. It is rich in vitamin E, another antioxidant, which helps protect one from cancer.

2. Sunflower Oil

Sunflower oil reduces the risk of cardiovascular diseases, fights free radicals (good for cancer patients) and is a healthy option for arthritis patients. Sunflower is an antioxidant. It prevents colon cancer, repairs the body, boosts the immune system and promotes proper functioning of the nervous system.

3. Groundnut Oil

Groundnut oil can boost energy and contains monounsaturated and polyunsaturated fats. It contains omega-3 fatty acids, lowers the risk of heart diseases and fights cancers, degenerative nerve disease, Alzheimer's disease and viral or fungal infections due to the presence of the antioxidant, resveratrol. On the flip side, groundnut oil tends to smoke at high temperatures.

4. Mustard Oil

Mustard oil, when consumed in moderation or sparingly, improves digestion and builds appetite. It also fights germs and viruses, and is great for preventing colds, coughs and skin problems.

5. Sesame Oil

Sesame oil is an edible oil extracted from sesame seeds. It is composed of polyunsaturated fatty acids like linoleic acid, monounsaturated fatty acids like oleic acid, and saturated fatty acids like palmitic acid, stearic acid, and others in small amounts.

Sesame oil has a high smoking point, which makes it suitable for sautéing, frying and deep frying.

Being rich in antioxidants, zinc, copper and calcium, it imparts health benefits like preventing cancer, improving heart health by keeping blood pressure in control, and reducing inflammation. It is excellent for skin and hair health and boosts bone density.

6. Edible Almond Oil

Almond oil is a light-coloured cooking oil used mostly in salads and vegetable dips. It is a superb source of vitamin E, is low in saturated (bad fats) and rich in monounsaturated fatty acids. It has health benefits like protecting our body from free radicals that cause cancer. It slows the ageing process, and reduces the risk of heart disease.

7. Palm Oil

Palm oil is an edible vegetable oil that is high in saturated fats and is derived from the fruit of the oil palm tree.

8. Soybean Oil

Soybean oil is extracted from soybean seeds. The major unsaturated fatty acids in it are polyunsaturated acids like alpha-linolenic acid and linoleic acid, monounsaturated fatty acids like oleic acid and saturated fatty acids like stearic acid and palmitic acid. Rich in phytosterol, it ensures reduction in blood cholesterol levels, and the vitamin E in it maintains the integrity of cell membrane and skin by protecting them from harmful free radicals. The vitamin K in it protects the brain from neuronal damage and acts as a great treatment for patients with Alzheimer's disease.

9. Canola Oil

Canola oil is extracted from rapeseed and is considered to be one of the healthiest oils known. It is low in saturated fats and high in omega-3 fatty acids. Replete with vitamin E, it is an antioxidant that fights free radical damage, thereby protecting you from cancer, and reducing the risk of heart disease and memory loss.

From Spices to Salt

Spices are made from dried fruits, seeds, barks or roots of certain plants. Some spices are used as flavouring agents while others impart a distinctive aroma to the dish to which they are added. The stage of cooking at which the spice is added is crucial to the flavour and aroma it produces in the dish. Spices get their aroma and flavour from the essential oils and chemical compounds present in them. It is necessary that these oils and compounds be released into the dish for it to acquire the spice's taste and aroma. This can be done either by grinding, grating, pounding or cooking the spices.

Spices that give flavour need to be added in the initial stages of cooking so that they release their flavours, while spices that are used for their aroma should be added at the end stage of cooking.

According to Ayurveda, spices can be warming or cooling, and are used to affect the balance of the digestive system. 'They act as a stimulus to the digestive system and relieve digestive disorders, and some spices are of antiseptic value,' explains Dr Krishnapura Srinivasan, a scientist at the Central Food Technological Research Institute in Mysore, India.

It is not surprising that spices have become associated with dieting.

'Spices are the most anti-oxidizing foods on the planet; they're very powerful foods,' says Gurpareet Bains, author of *Indian Superspices*, a collection of 'lab-inspired' recipes designed to treat the symptoms of everyday illnesses. 'Everyone says that Indian food is unhealthy, but with *Indian Superspices*, I completely throw that out of the window because Indian food can be medicine at the same time.'

Turmeric

Every year, we bring fresh underground turmeric stems (rhizomes), dry them in bright sunlight, and powder them to store for the rest of the year. Turmeric, with its bright yellow colour, and due to the presence of the powerful polyphenol, curcumin, imparts various health benefits. The first of which is its ability to fight dangerous diseases like cancer, atherosclerosis and neuro-degenerative diseases. Its anti-bacterial and anti-fungal properties make it very effective when it comes to common health complaints like cold, cough and sore throat. Minor cuts and burns can be treated simply by applying some turmeric to them, thanks to its antiseptic properties.

Fennel

Armed with phytonutrients and antioxidants, cancer cells have to accept defeat when faced with fennel. Anethole, a major constituent of fennel, resists and restricts the adhesive and invasive activities of cancer cells. It suppresses the enzymatic, regulated activities that cause cancer cell multiplication. A tomato fennel soup with garlic or fresh salads with fennel bulbs make for an ideal entree prior to an elaborate course meal. Roasted fennel with parmesan can be another star pick.

Not Only Mouth-fresheners

I discovered fennel (saunf) after Viaan's birth. I was told to have it boiled in water, which I stored in a flask and sipped throughout the day as it is great for lactation and prevents the child from getting colicky. I liked the taste and after-effects so much that I continue to have it.

I discovered a new antidote for acidity. Mix half a spoon of roasted ajwain and half a spoon of roasted fennel seeds in water, boil for fifteen minutes, strain and sip on it like tea.

That's why its served at the end at Indian meals as it is a digestive. You should avoid the kind that is coated with sugar, though, because doign so kills the digestive purpose. Just plain, roasted, good old saunf rocks!

Saffron

Saffron contains a natural carotenoid dicarboxylic acid called crocetin; it is an effective cancer-fighting element. It not only inhibits the progression of the disease but also decreases the size of the tumour by half, guaranteeing a complete cure. Though it is the most expensive spice in the world, because around 250,000 flower stigmas of the saffron crocus make just about half a kilo, even a few saffron threads are sufficient to avail the benefits of saffron, for which you won't regret paying for.

Cumin

Cumin aids digestion, which is probably why we like chewing cumin seeds at the end of every meal. However, its health benefits go beyond digestion. A potent herb with antioxidant characteristics, cumin contains a compound called thymoquinone, which checks the proliferation of cells responsible for prostate cancer. So instead of loading your usual snack options with calories and oil, add this seasoning to your bread, fried beans or sauce, and make the dish rich in flavour and high in health. You can rediscover the magic of cumin in your regular bowl of tadka dal and rice too.

Cinnamon

It takes not more than half a teaspoon of cinnamon powder every day to keep the risk of cancer away. A natural food preservative, cinnamon is a source of iron and calcium. Useful in reducing tumour growth, it blocks the formation of new vessels in the human body. Some of the effective ways of including cinnamon in your diet are as follows:

- Start your day with a cup of cinnamon tea (leaves or sachets)
- Add this wonder spice to your morning oatmeal

- Prepare a fruity delight comprising chopped apples, a few walnuts and cinnamon
- Honey and cinnamon in your glass of milk before going to bed is also a wonderful option

Oregano

More than a pizza or pasta topping, oregano confirms its worth as a potential agent against prostate cancer. Consisting of antimicrobial compounds, just one teaspoon of oregano has the power of two cups of red grapes! Phytochemical quercetin present in oregano restricts growth of malignant cells in the body and acts like a drug against cancers.

Heeng (Asafoetida)

Though it doesn't have its origin in India, heeng is widely used in Indian cooking. It is ochre in colour and has a strong, pungent aroma. It is highly recommended for people with indigestion, stomach upsets, bloating, flatulence and intestinal gas. You can add half a teaspoon of heeng to water or buttermilk to get instant relief in case of any digestive problem. In India, a pinch of heeng is used in food that is consumed daily, like sabzi, dal, gravies, sambhar, and so on. If you do not use heeng yet, it is advisable to begin right away.

Elaichi

The most aromatic of all Indian spices, our very own elaichi is consumed in two forms—choti elaichi (green pods) and badi elaichi (black pods). Bad breath, loss of appetite, depression, indigestion, nausea; you name it, and cardamom cures it. It is a great carminative (causing expulsion of gas), diuretic (causing urination), digestive, expectorant (helps bring up phlegm from the lungs) and stimulant. Apart from its health benefits, who can do without a cup of hot elaichi chai?

Cloves

These dried flower buds of the clove tree are considered one of the 'hottest' among spices. They have anti-bacterial and antiseptic properties. Being a natural anaesthetic, it has been used as a remedy for toothache for ages.

Black Pepper

Black pepper is the fruit of the black pepper plant from the Piperaceae family. It has a pungent taste which is due to the alkaloid, chavicine. It helps relieve symptoms of common cold. You can add black pepper to your hot vegetable soup and enjoy it when you have a cold.

Methi (Fenugreek)

Methi seeds are tiny, light brown in colour, and are bitter to taste. They are used in particular recipes like kadhi, as well as in various curries. Special ladoos with methi are prepared for pregnant and lactating mothers to ease the process of delivery and stimulate the production of breast milk. Methi seeds can be soaked overnight and consumed early in the morning to stabilize blood sugar, reduce cholesterol levels, and flush out toxins from body.

Shilpa's Tips

My grandma had a methi seed trick. This is great to ferment idlis and dhoklas, as a healthier option instead of soda or yeast. Add to the batter one tablespoon of powdered methi seeds and toddy or nariyal pani (tender coconut water). See how fluffy and sweet your idlis turn out.

Red Chilli Powder

In Indian food, we use both red and green chillies. Chillies have a strong, spicy taste that tingles your taste buds because of the active alkaloid compound, capsaicin, present in it. Chillies are rich in vitamins A and C, and hence are excellent antioxidants. They build up immunity and fight off free radicals responsible for cancerous growth. Chillies are also known to be good sources of minerals like iron, potassium and magnesium. Research shows that to some extent, chillies also help reduce the bad cholesterol (LDL). However, if consumed in excess, they can cause inflammation. People suffering from any type of gastrointestinal problems should avoid chillies.

Legumes

Legumes are plants which produce pods with seeds. They can be classified into the following types:

- Lentils: These are tiny, round and flat seeds which are known as 'dal' in India. These include red lentils, brown lentils, black lentils, french lentils, and so on. Lentils are available in the market in two forms: whole and split. For example, moong is of two kinds, whole (green gram) and split (yellow moong).

- Beans: Beans are neither fruit nor vegetable but are seeds which are used as food to eat. Examples of beans include kidney beans, moth beans, soybean, and so on.
- Peas: Peas are spherical green seeds which are eaten as a vegetable.
- Peanuts: Peanuts develop in pods which ripen underground.

Legumes are good sources of carbohydrates, proteins, fibre, and are low in fat. They are packed with calcium, iron, folate, magnesium, potassium, zinc, vitamin B_6, thiamin and riboflavin. They are easy to cook and store, and can be cooked in diverse ways. With a base sauce of onion and tomato, ginger and garlic, various dishes like curries, soups, parathas etc. can be prepared with legumes.

When I don't have any vegetable to cook, lentils are the quickest option to prepare. You just need to soak them and then cook them with your favourite ingredients and in your style.

Health Benefits of Legumes

Legumes mentioned above are rich in carbohydrates, proteins, fibre and minerals like folate and magnesium. Each of these plays an improtant role in the body.

- The complex carbohydrates in legumes make one feel charged up throughout the day because they release energy slowly and steadily.
- For vegetarians, lentils are a good source of protein, and help them build up muscle to get a lean and toned body.
- Fibre in lentils playes various roles, such as:
    1. It binds with carbohydrates in food, slowing digestion and stabilizing blood sugar levels.
    2. It binds with the fats and cholesterols in the foods and help regulate cholesterol levels. This aids in reducing the risk of heart attacks by clearing out arteries.
    3. The soluble fibre in lentils absorbs water, forms gels and relieves digestive problems like constipation, irritable bowel syndrome and diverticulitis.
    4. The high fibre content of lentils keeps the food for a longer time in the digestive tract, making you feel full.
- Folate and magnesium present in lentils have a special role to play in maintaining heart health. Folate lowers the levels of homocysteine in blood which is responsible for damaging arteries and putting you at the risk of heart disease. Magnesium improves the flow of blood, oxygen and nutrients throughout the body.

How to Consume Legumes

Having discussed the benefits of legumes, one must also remember that anything in excess can be toxic.

People avoid eating legumes for various reasons. The most commonly heard is that it leads to digestive issues like flatulence and bloating. By taking certain steps, we can enjoy eating legumes more often.

Phytic Acids

Pulses contain phytic acids which interfere with the absorption of iron, zinc and magnesium and can result in mineral deficiencies. Soaking, sprouting and fermentation will help reduce the phytate content of legumes.

Lectins in pulses resist digestion, which can also lead to flatulence and bloating. Soaking legumes overnight and cooking them properly will reduce their lectin content, thereby allowing for their proper digestion.

Develop the habit of chewing your food thoroughly so that the process of digesting legumes can start in your mouth.

At times people stop consuming proteins, including legumes, because the purines in proteins increase uric acid levels in the body, which can lead to diseases like gout. Other health consequences might be flatulence and an overload on the kidneys. Except a few beans, you can include lentils and split dals in your diet. Just remember to hydrate properly to flush out uric acid from the body.

Most recipes in Indian cuisine make use of legumes, lentils and cereals. There are many Indian recipes that call for soaking the legumes, lentils, nuts and cereals in water prior to cooking them. It's important to do so, otherwise they take a long time to cook. For instance, whenever we prepare rajma, chana or chhole, we soak them overnight in water. However, it's not absolutely necessary to soak them, as even without soaking, cooking takes fifteen to twenty minutes.

Although, legumes, cereals and lentils are rich in nutrients and enzymes, they also contain phytic acid, which is a type of a phosphorous compound that inhibits the absorption of important minerals like calcium, magnesium, iron, copper and zinc. Actually, phytic acid is a way for nature to protect the seed until the conditions for it to sprout and grow arise. In addition to blocking key minerals from being absorbed into the body, phytic acid places a great strain on the human digestive system. Traditionally, people have soaked and sprouted seeds, nuts, legumes and grains in order to derive optimal nutritional benefits. Once soaked, phytic acid is deactivated and released into the water, and the enzymes and minerals in the food are more readily available for absorption into our bodies.

Fibre

Dietary fibre or roughage is the indigestible portion of food derived from plants. The recommended daily intake of fibre for adults is around 20 to 35 grams.

There are two types of fibre: soluble and insoluble.

Soluble Fibre: Soluble fibre includes pectins, gums, mucilages, and some hemicelluloses. As the name suggests, these are soluble in some medium. Soluble fibre gets dissolved in water from food or the digestive juices to form a viscous liquid or gel. This gel binds with certain food components and makes them unavailable for absorption. This property of soluble fibres makes them useful for several health reasons:

1. Cholesterol binds with this gel and is eliminated from the body, thus reducing the chances of heart-related risk factors.
2. Diabetes is kept in check as soluble fibres slow down the entrance of glucose into the bloodstream, thereby preventing spikes in blood glucose and insulin.
3. The gel binds with food components in the stomach, making them pass slowly through the digestive tract. This aids in weight loss because it makes one feel full for a longer period of time and helps prevent overeating.
4. Soluble fibre soaks water and makes stools bulkier, thereby relieving digestive problems like constipation and diarrhoea.

Good sources of soluble fibre include oats, legumes (peas, beans, lentils), barley, fruits and vegetables (especially oranges, apples and carrots).

Insoluble Fibre: Cellulose, lignins, and some hemicelluloses are insoluble fibres. They do not dissolve in water and hence travel through the digestive system in their original form. They have a curative effect on bowel-related problems like constipation and piles, and aid in regular bowel movements.

Sources include whole wheat flour, wheat bran, nuts, beans and vegetables like cauliflower and green beans.

How to increase fibre in your diet:

1. Replace refined products like refined wheat flour, pasta and processed foods with whole cereals like whole wheat flour, jowar, bajra, ragi and brown rice.
2. Instead of juices, consume whole fruit and vegetables like pear, strawberries, apples, carrots, cabbage, broccoli, and so on.
3. Snack on high fibre munchies like fruits, vegetables and nuts to pacify mid-morning and evening hunger pangs.
4. Choose legumes, beans or pulses in place of meat.
5. Consume isabgol (psyllium husk) regularly.

Note: Do not forget to hydrate yourself properly after consuming high fibre foods to reap the maximum benefit.

Salt

Salt is an indispensable ingredient in all cooked food, except desserts, of course. It is essential to impart flavour to food, and is also used as a preservative. Be it hot and spicy North Indian cuisine, or West Indian cuisine that imbibes a touch of sweetness in all its dishes, the famous dosa and idli of South India, or the delicious food of East India, salt is the one common ingredient in all these cuisines.

The element sodium binds with chlorine to form sodium chloride, or what is commonly known as 'table salt'. The American Heart Association recommends that we limit our sodium intake to not more than 2,300 mg per day for the general population and 1,500 mg per day for hypertensive individuals. We can easily get the required amount of salt from food. In fact, we end up eating more salt than we require because of our increased consumption of processed and packaged foods which is loaded with sodium.

There are three kinds of salt available in the market:

1. Sea Salt: This is made after evaporating ocean salt or salt water lakes and involves very little processing. This ensures the salt retains most of its nutrients.
2. Rock salt: Also known as halite, it is the mineral form of sodium chloride.
3. Table salt: It is the most processed salt from which all natural nutrients have been washed away.

Comparing sea salt with table salt is similar to comparing sugarcane juice with sugar. You will always hear doctors and nutritionists encouraging you to have sugarcane juice but avoid sugar. This is because sugarcane juice is not processed and retains most of inutrients but when it is processed to obtain sugar, all these nutrients are lost.

Salt is rich in sodium and also contains magnesium and potassium. Magnesium and potassium work hand in hand with sodium to maintain the water balance in the body. But nowadays, due to the increased availability and consumption of processed, packaged and canned foods in the market, one's sodium intake can be in excess of what is needed. This leads to an imbalance in the amounts of sodium vis-a-vis magnesium and potassium, leading to a greater risk to one's health.

In places like Galicia in north-west Spain, Japan, and the US, the high consumption of iodine found in iodized salt is known to cause hyperthyroidism, where the production of thyroid hormone increases above normal levels. This leads to weight loss, fatigue, hyperactivity, increased heart rate and blood pressure, abnormal heart rhythm (arrhythmia), excessive sweating, shakiness of hands and insomnia.

This should make one cautious about the kind of salt one buys from the market. Don't just check the labels of foods that contain sugar, fats or fibre, but also the labels on packets of salt. If the label says only 'sodium chloride', put it back on the shelf and move on.

Along with checking the label on the salt packet, one should also check its colour. Its colour will guide us towards the best salt to pick up. We know that salt is white in colour and hence will tend to choose the whitest salt on the shelf. However it would be useful to remember that unrefined salt can contain more that ninety trace elements and its colour is not pure white. For instance, sea salt will contain microscopic amounts of sea life, which provide natural iodine. It is grey in colour and even a little moist, indicating high mineral content.

Benefits of Sea Salt

The major nutrients present in sea salt are sodium, potassium, magnesium, silicon, phosphorus and calcium. Its benefits include:

S- Skin care
E- Effective for aching feet

A- Alkalizing
S- Strong immune system
A- Aids weight loss
L- Lets you be stress free
T- Total health care

Skin care: Sea salt, being rich is magnesium, is known to open up skin pores and flush out toxins, thus improving blood circulation and hydrating the skin to keep it healthy. By keeping the skin moist, sea salt provides relief from dry and itchy skin and is a good treatment for certain skin diseases like psoriasis and eczema.

Effective for aching feet: The best solution for your tired feet, or for people with muscular soreness after a long run or workout, is to soak your feet in lukewarm water with sea salt added to it. It relaxes the feet and relieves pain.

Alkalizing: Sea salt is rich in sodium, potassium and other minerals which help make the body alkaline.

Strong immune system: Because of the alkalizing effect of sea salt on the body, bacteria and viruses are not able to thrive. This ensures a boost to the body's immunity.

Aids weight loss: With a high consumption of saturated fats, sugar and excess proteins, our digestive system becomes sluggish as the food sticks to the intestinal lining, particularly the colon. A sea salt cleanse helps flush out the toxins, kickstart the digestive system and the metabolism, and aid in weight loss.

Lots you be stress free: Research has shown that sea salt helps in the production of serotonin (the 'feel good hormone') and melatonin (the 'relaxing hormone'). It calms your mind and helps you sleep well.

Total health care: If you club together the benefits of sea salt, you realize how important it is to keep your body free from disease. It helps keep your cholesterol levels in check, blood pressure normal, reduces the risk of heart disease, stabilizes blood sugar, prevents diabetes, and even reduces inflammation of the respiratory tract, thus helping people with asthma breathe better.

Calcium and Vitamin D

With changing lifestyles, lack of exercise and proper nutrition, osteoporosis is increasingly affecting the lives of women in their youth, middle age, and pre- and post-menopause. Many think that just getting enough calcium is sufficient, but there is more to it than that. To prevent or improve osteoporosis, you need to consider the following factors:

- Calcium
- Vitamin D
- Weight-bearing exercises
- Hormone replacement through medication or natural foods

If you do not get enough calcium because you do not consume enough of the foods in the above list, you may be popping supplements that contain 1,200 mg of calcium per day, but do remember that calcium gets absorbed into the body only in the presence of vitamin D. So, if your vitamin D levels are low, chances are that no matter how much calcium you take, it will not be absorbed into your body.

Foods Rich in Calcium

Tofu
Soya milk
Soybean
Turnip
Okra
Sweet lime
Broccoli
Almond
Cabbage
Dark green, leafy vegetables
Peas
Milk
Cheese
Yoghurt
Beans
Chickpea
Orange
Figs
Raisins
Sesame
Bell pepper

This is the answer to the often asked question, 'Why do my bones hurt when I'm popping calcium supplements every day?' On further investigation, we have noticed that vitamin D levels are often extremely low, especially among vegetarians.

You get vitamin D only from sunshine and fortified foods, or vitamin D supplements. Our body is not capable of making this vitamin. Fish oils are a rich source of vitamin D as a non-vegetarian option. Taking a vitamin D shot under a doctor's supervision will also take care of its deficiency.

Among women who have had their ovaries removed, low oestrogen production might lead to osteoporosis. They should maintain a daily intake of 1,200 mg of calcium, ensure their vitamin D levels are high, and should also get more sunshine and do weight-bearing exercises.

In certain cases, hormone replacement through natural foods is used to reverse this condition and help the body produce oestrogen.

To do weight-bearing exercises, you do not have to go to the gym. These exercises involve the use of your own body weight and include walking, swimming, aerobics, dancing, tennis, weight training, cross-country running and gymnastics.

In case you already suffer from osteoporosis, and exercising is hard on your bones, try to swim or work out in water. This will take the pressure off your bones and joints, and strengthen them at the same time.

The following are ways in which you could prevent or improve this condition:

- Check your calcium and vitamin D intake and levels.
- Get sunshine whenever possible.
- Eat calcium-rich foods.
- Exercise for thirty to forty minutes at least four to six times a week.

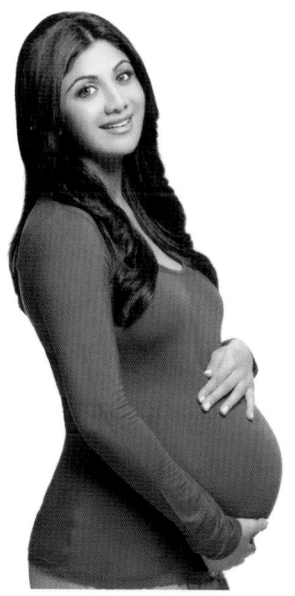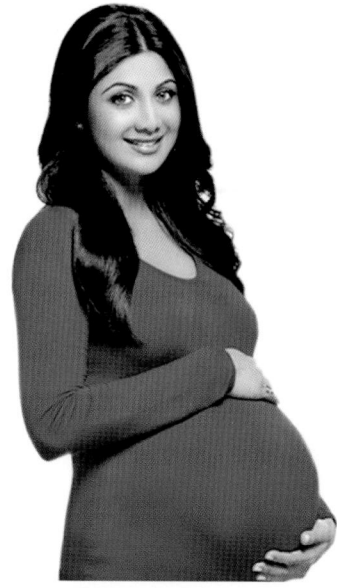

During pregnancy with my baby bump

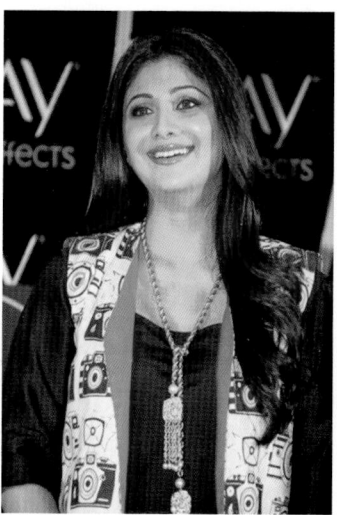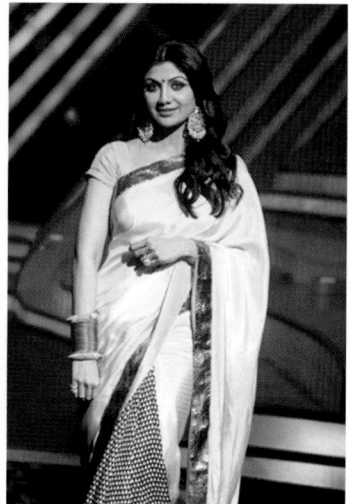

After pregnancy when I had put on 32 kilos

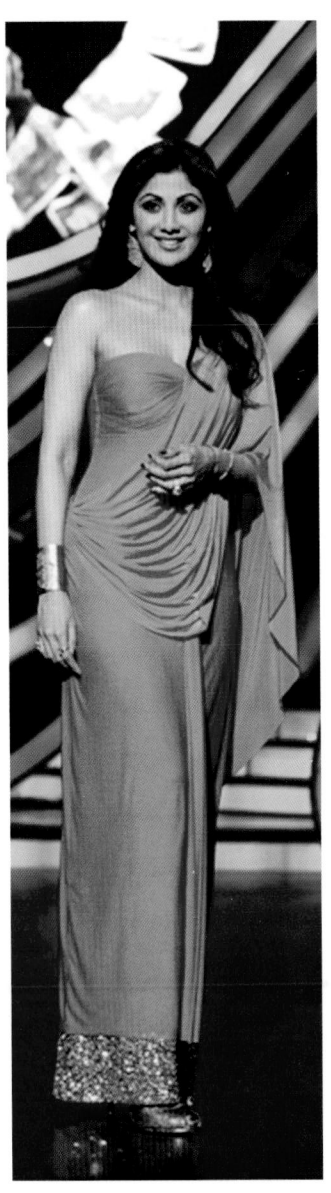

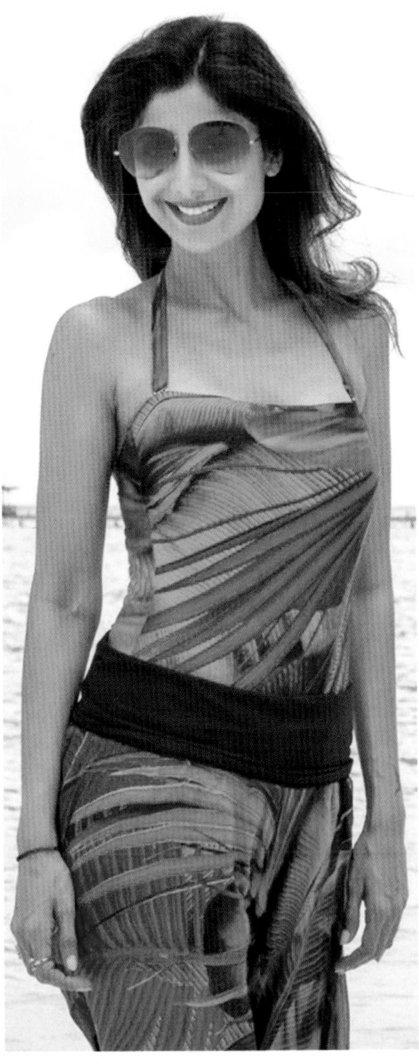

After losing 32 kilos

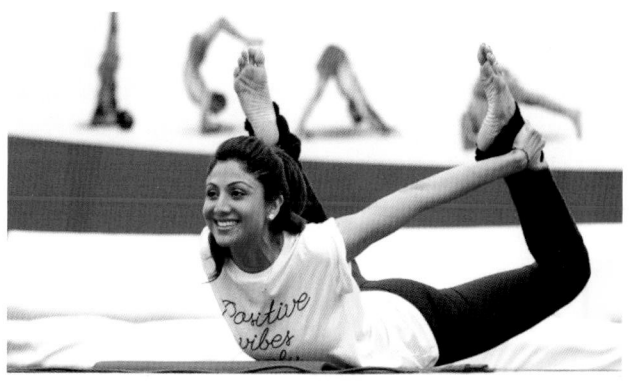

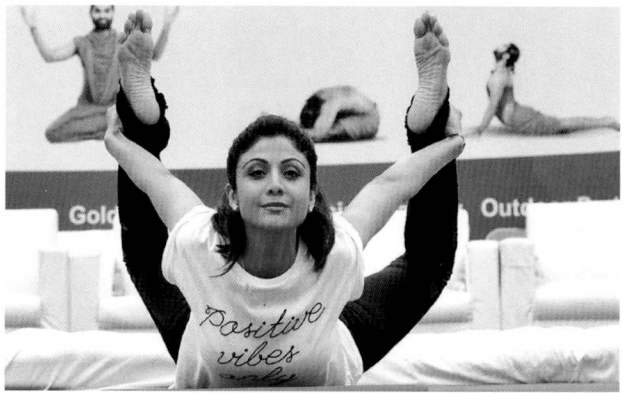

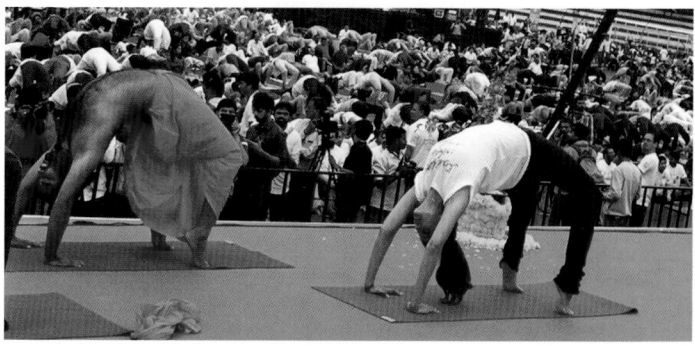

Following my other passion while demonstrating yoga poses on
World Yoga Day in Bengaluru with 12,000 people

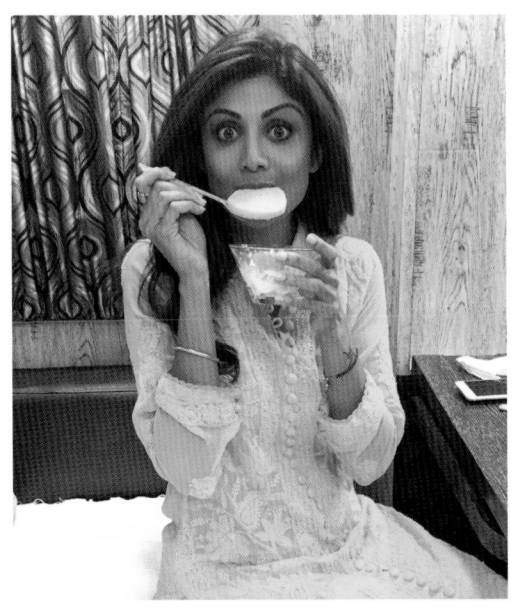

My Sunday binge spree; gorging on yummy malai kulfi

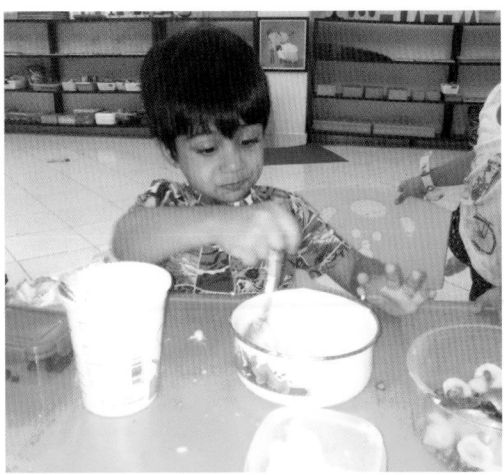

Encourage children to have fun with healthy foods;
my son Viaan making a fruit salad with yoghurt

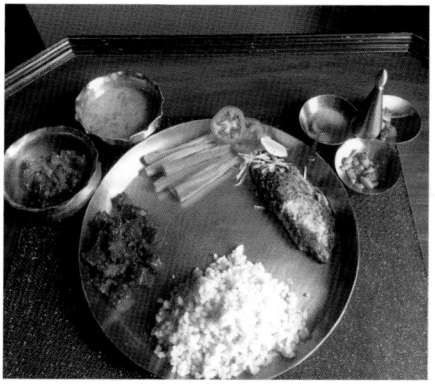

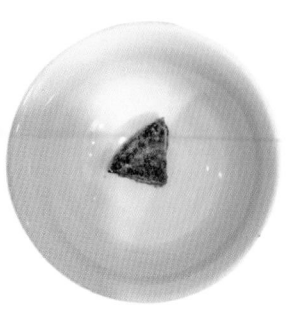

My ideal lunch of red rice, dal, a piece of grilled mint fish, beetroot sabzi, baigan bharta, carrots with ghee and pickles

The piece of black jaggery I have after lunch (3–4 times a week)

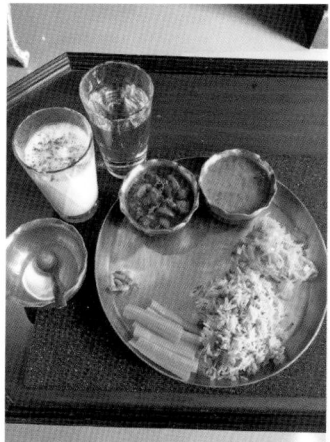

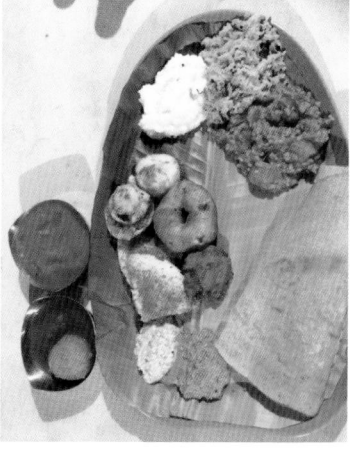

My simple lunch. Jeera and rock salt chaas (skimmed-milk yoghurt), ghee, garlic (homemade) pickle, mushroom curry, cabbage, two carrots, veg pulao (brown rice)

My favourite South Indian fare; who says healthy food can't be tasty?

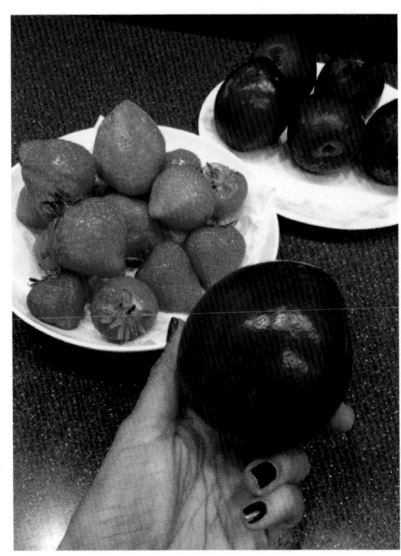

My favourite fruits, the luscious strawberries and plums

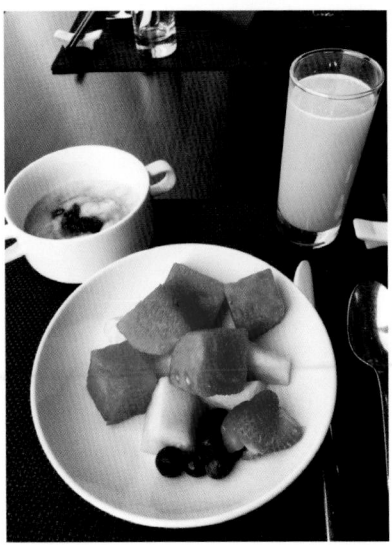

Porridge in water with honey and raisins; pineapple and watermelon
with freshly squeezed orange juice

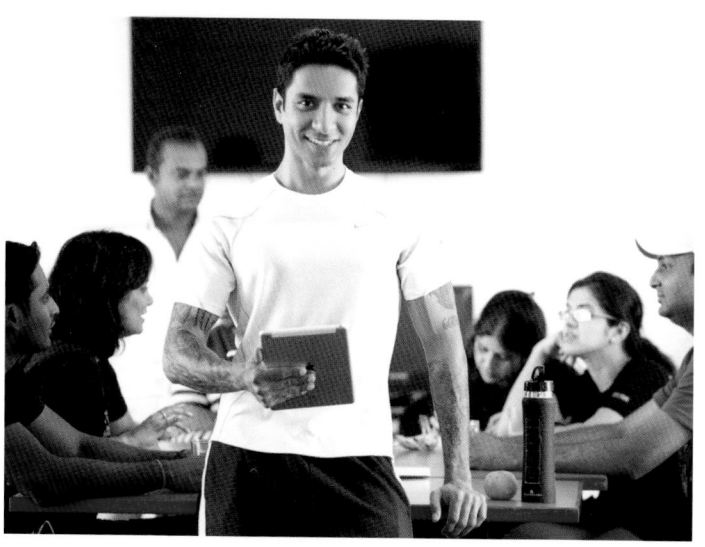

Luke Coutinho, the co-author

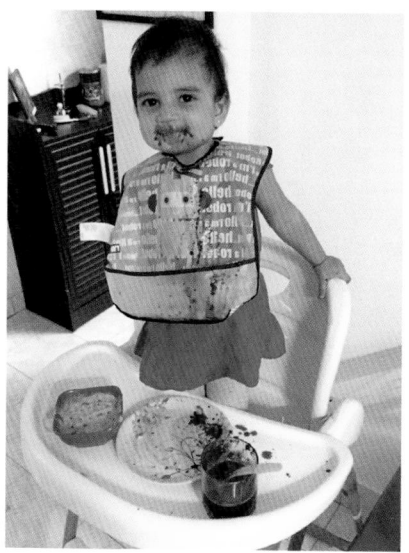

Luke's daughter, Tyanna, having dal and curd with a
mixed vegetable raw juice with Indian spices and coconut oil

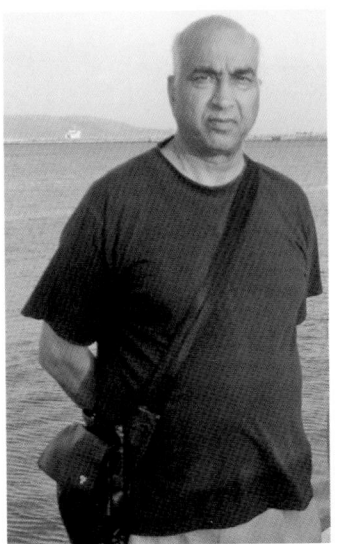
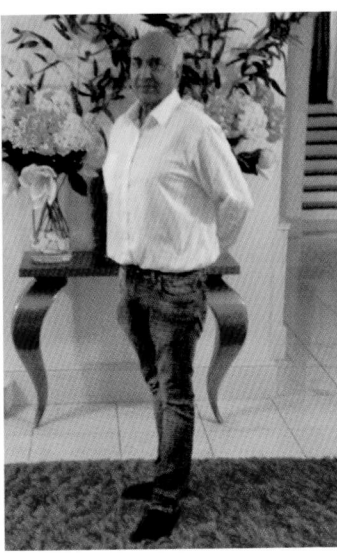

My father-in-law, Balkrishan Kundra, who lost 13 kilos in six weeks

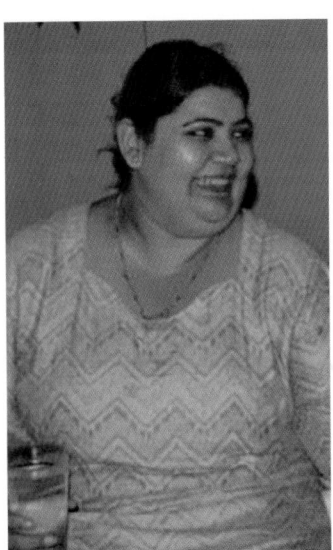
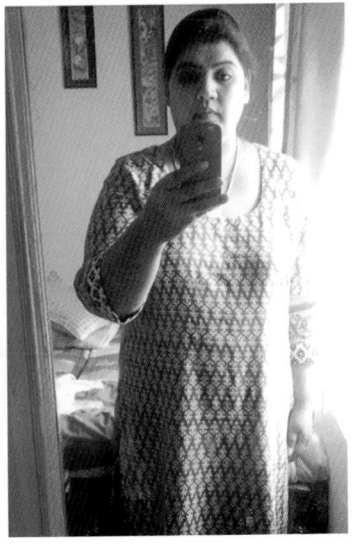

Aarti who lost 22 kilos in seven months after consulting with Luke

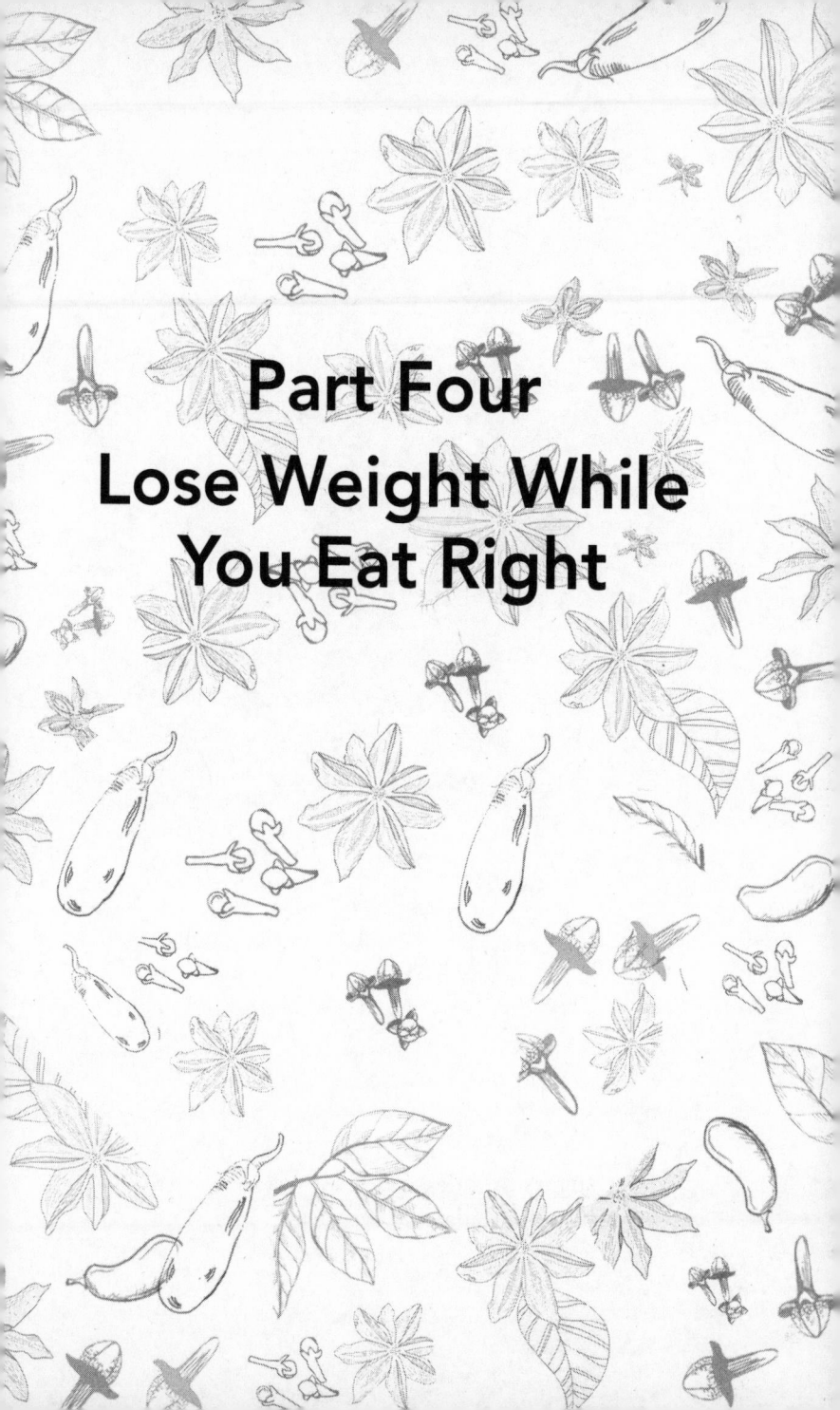

Part Four
Lose Weight While You Eat Right

Understanding and Eliminating Fat

Why do we get fat? To answer this question, it is extremely important to understand the concept of fat and how it builds up in the body. Irrespective of whatever world cuisine or food you eat, the principle remains the same. When you understand this simple concept, you would have begun your journey to healthy and easy fat loss.

In a landmark study, researchers from Boston discovered that people who have high insulin levels have a more difficult time losing weight than people who have low levels of insulin. When people don't eat the right foods, the body automatically makes an adjustment to deal with the sugar and unnatural ingredients being consumed. The only way the body can adjust is to produce more insulin. So, the body becomes an insulin-producing machine. Once the body releases insulin, it is unable to burn fat. So, the key to having the body burn fat like it is supposed to, is to have low levels of insulin and eat the right foods.

How to Make Sense of All the Information Around?

If you are one of those people who have struggled for most of your life with your weight, you are not alone. If you are struggling to lose weight, I understand how you feel. Many men and women have tried to lose weight but have failed. Let's face it. Losing weight can be difficult. Why? There are various reasons for obesity, including addiction to food, little or no exercise, stress, and lack of knowledge about the right foods to eat.

One of the problems we face today is that there is a lot of confusion about the best foods to eat and what foods actually burn body fat. Many Indian foods, especially whole grains, lentils, legumes, nuts, lean meats, vegetables, and healthy fats do not rapidly spike insulin levels, and instead convert your body into a fat-burning machine. For example, most people falsely believe that they should only be eating egg whites and not the yolk when they're trying to be healthy and lose weight. Nothing could be further from the truth! In fact, over 99 per cent of the important vitamins, minerals and nutrients are found in the yolk of the egg, and not in the white. A recent study published in the *Journal of the American College of Nutrition* found that when people ate two eggs for breakfast, they consumed about four hundred fewer calories over the next twenty-four hours! That means you can have a great breakfast and lose more weight because the nutrients in the yolk help control your appetite and burn body fat.

When people have applied these simple principles, they have been able to significantly boost their metabolisms and automatically put their bodies in fat-burning mode.

They were also able to automatically improve every other aspect of their health, including more energy, a flat stomach, greater confidence, a toned body, and even better sex drive!

The honest truth, as I've said before, is that there are no secrets when it comes to losing weight or a diet plan. The only way to lose weight is with discipline. I know I'm harping on this but there is a reason: **weight and discipline are directly proportional to each other.**

The fact is that most plans on the market are simply fads. They don't really work. You may end up losing weight, only to gain it right back.

So, is there no hope? Of course there is. If you want to lose weight and sustain it, you need to make changes in your lifestyle, as well as follow the right diet. You can get rid of excess body fat, but the change starts with you. It starts with your attitude. Always remember that it's mind over body.

You may have developed poor dietary habits and hence gained weight. Whether you know it or not, your mental state does have a lot to do with your body size and percentage of body fat. You have to look in the mirror and decide how you want to look. Do you want to be obese or do you want to look slim and fit? It takes determination and a strong desire to be successful to lose weight and get the healthy body you have always wanted.

Let's take the real-life example of Neha. Neha is twenty-eight and has had trouble with her weight. She tried several diets, only to go back to being overweight. She tried nearly everything, including hypnosis. But she always ended up regaining any weight she lost. Why? It was because of her habit of eating junk food, which she would go back to between the diets. That is all she knew about eating. She would often cheat and eat fried chicken, French fries, doughnuts, potato chips and so on. She did this on a regular basis.

On the other hand, there is Devyani, a thirty-two-year-old IT professional. She had been slim most of her life, until she got married. Her father was a nutritionist, and her mother worked as a nurse. So, growing up, she had a healthy lifestyle. However her husband had grown up eating junk food. So, when they got married, Devyani began to eat what her husband did. A year later, she had gained nearly 20 kilos. One day, she looked at herself in the mirror and began to cry. She knew she had to do something. So, she tried an experiment. She prepared his food one way and hers the way she had before marriage.

After doing this for a month, she lost 4 kilos! Her husband noticed it and decided to try her way of eating. Within two weeks, he felt better, had more energy, and even began to lose weight. Some people visualize themselves as slim and healthy, and achieve that. If you have never done this before, perhaps you might want to consider it now. Picturing the outcome will help you get to that point. This is the important bit, called the art of visual manifestation. Visualize how you want to be, and that will become reality. You are the architect of your own health.

One good way for you to lose weight is by setting goals. Those who have set goals have found that life is more manageable for them, and they are able to lose weight and gain a healthy body. Whatever you do, don't make excuses for why you are overweight. Instead, create a mindset for success. You have to understand why it matters what you eat. Keep reading, and you will learn why.

How You Got Fat

Anything you do starts in your mind. This is where your thinking process begins. So, if you take a step back and look at your life, you will probably recall when your weight problems actually started.

For many people, the weight problems began when they ate more junk food than they wished to. They liked certain foods and so they kept eating them. The result was obvious.

Many perhaps fell for the lies and deceptions that the food industry has been feeding us for so long. Or perhaps they hated facing certain emotions. You will be surprised how many people go to counselling, join a twelve-step programme or seek a psychologist to help them with their food addictions.

This could be true for anybody who is overweight. Or there might be a totally different trigger for putting on weight. One should definitely be aware that there is a problem, and why it exists.

Read on to find out why people gain weight. It may just be an eye-opener.

Reasons Why People May Be Overweight

- Perhaps you work full-time and just don't have the time to cook. So, you buy ready-made dinners that are processed or use refined ingredients that give them a longer shelf life.

- A person's metabolism might be the main cause. Some people can eat huge amounts and not gain an ounce, while some who eat very little pile on the kilos. If you are unsure of what I am referring to, think of a car engine. If your engine is running at an idle speed, it is burning an even amount of gas. The rate of burn will be slow and steady. But the minute you step on the gas, the engine is fed a lot more gas to allow for a greater burning of fuel. Your body does the same thing. When your body is at rest is your basal metabolic rate (BMR). Some people have a fast BMR, while others have a slow one. This is due to the foods you eat, because some foods actually increase your metabolism and turn your body into a fat-burning machine and other foods slow down your metabolism and cause it to be in fat-storing mode. Those who have a fast BMR are able to burn a lot of calories right away. This is why they never gain weight. For those with a slow BMR, the results are often apparent in the form of weight gain despite not eating very much.
- Over-consumption of hydrogenated fats, trans fats and saturated fats leads to these being deposited on your body, especially the abdominal area. This leads to belly fat that is often quite difficult to get rid of.

You see, the body cannot discern the amounts of calories it is consuming. It will only gauge the amount of food you put in it. Whatever extra calories your eat will be stored in your body as fat. The bottom line is that you control not only the kind of foods you eat, but also the amount of food you eat. The best way to do this is to ignore what the food industry tells you about the foods you must eat, and avoid the junk food you find in stores and fast food restaurants. We'll talk more about what not to eat and what to eat later. Right now, let's understand why it is so important for you to eat the right foods.

Why the Right Diet Works: Technique and Logic

If you want to lose body fat, you need to modify the way you eat. There is no way around it.

If you want to lose excess weight and become healthy, you need to learn how to eat foods to speed up your metabolism and turn your body into a fat-burning machine. Everything you put in your mouth will do something to your body; it will either burn fat or store fat.

How does this happen? The human body is a chemical-producing machine with cells that can multiply and divide. When you feed your body certain foods, these are broken down in the stomach and digested. The digested matter is then taken apart and used by the body for various purposes. It is for this reason that you have to be careful what you put in your mouth. When you eat processed or refined foods, the body does not know what to do with it. Most processed junk food does not get used and is stored in the body as fat. For example, if you are eating a lot of junk food, you will probably find you have a lot of energy at first, but will crash a little later. You also notice your clothes getting tighter.

When you eat healthy, you also feel healthy. For e.g., how do you feel when you gulp down a can of coke?

You certainly feel great at the time, but later start feeling heaviness in the stomach and feel guilty too for having made that unhealthy choice. Instead, when you ignore that can of coke and sip on lemon water, you may feel deprived at the time but at the back of your mind, you feel great because you have assured yourself of an excellent source of energy which is going to help detoxify your body and will not get stored as fat.

When you start eating the right foods, within a reasonable time, you'll feel like a million bucks. You will feel energized, your sex life will take a turn for the better, and you'll feel youthful!

Lose Weight with the Great Indian Diet

Before we go into how you can turn your body into a fat-burning machine, I would like to address how your body handles the foods you eat. This way, you will have a better understanding as to what happens to foods in your body.

When you eat, there are processes that begin at digestion. Certain hormones kick in and direct the body to use what you eat in certain ways. The one hormone our body uses most frequently during digestion is insulin.

When people hear the word 'insulin', they automatically think of diabetes and sugar problems. This is not always the case. Insulin is an anabolic hormone that takes the nutrients from the foods we eat and transfers them to our muscle cells. If we were inside our bodies, we would see a complex mechanism at work, doing wonders that we could never comprehend. For instance, when we eat carbohydrates, our system breaks them down and sends some of the nutrients to our bloodstream, thereby raising the blood sugar level. Then, the pancreas secretes insulin to counter the excess sugar injected into the blood and converts it into fat, muscle glycogen, or liver glycogen. If your muscle or liver glycogen levels are already maxed out, the excess blood sugar will be stored as fat.

If, during this period, you work out properly and regularly, your body will take the excess sugar that was stored as fat and transfer it to muscle glycogen to be used by your muscle cells. If you eat protein along with foods that contains fibre, this can slow down or speed up your digestion. It depends on the amount of protein and fibre, as well as the other fats you consume. The more protein, fibre and fats you eat with the carbohydrates, the slower the carbohydrates will be digested. This will raise your blood sugar level slowly and steadily. Hence, the release of insulin will also be slower.

If on eating carbohydrates, you experience a boost of energy only for it to crash soon after, it means your carbohydrates were digested quickly. Foods from which fibre has been removed can be digested faster. Any time such foods, like white bread, low-fibre cereals, candy and other high-sugar foods, are eaten, the person will experience a boost of energy, followed by a crash. It is for this reason that people who live on such a diet are constantly eating. They need that boost again and again. The result is stored body fat that makes you obese. Other foods that have been known to raise blood sugar quickly include white rice, sugars (except fructose), ice cream, candy and cakes. Any carbohydrates that have been refined and contain no fibre can be included in this list. On the other hand are foods that are slow to digest, and therefore do not raise blood sugar levels quickly, including most fruits and vegetables, sweet potatoes, barley, beans and most other high fibre carbohydrates.

Any kind of carbohydrate has to be consumed in combination with fibre. The ratio that should be maintained is 1.5 to 2 grams of fibre per every 10 grams of carbohydrates.

Now that you understand how the body uses what you eat, let's go over how you can turn your body into a fat-burning machine. The main thing you need to do is eat three meals a day—lunch being the biggest—and two snacks (nuts, fruit and fibre-rich food). If you are an early riser, then a heavier breakfast is advisable. It is fine to increase the volume of food you eat as long as you eat fat-burning foods. Also, drink plenty of water during the day. This helps flush out the system and get rid of impurities. If you have a salad, spread almond butter or hummus on the veggies instead of salad dressing. I will go into detail about these food items later. Your main consideration should be to control your insulin levels and watch your fat intake. As you consume omega-3 fatty acids from fish and grass-fed animals, you will find that it will work inside your body to burn any fat you have stored. The omega-3 fatty acid does this by interacting with cell receptors called PPARs, which stimulate the fat-burning genes.

Think about that for a second. You do have fat-burning genes in your body. You just need to activate them. You'll be amazed by what your body is capable of when you feed it the nutrients it needs. You will not only see the results, but will also feel the results.

Once you start eating fat-burning foods, within a day or two, you will begin to feel slimmer and lighter.

You may at first still have cravings for junk food. This is normal. This may be because your body is going through junk food withdrawal, and your body is addicted to it. But this withdrawal process will only last for two or three weeks. The key here is to stick to eating only fat-burning foods through this withdrawal period. After that, it will be easy, and you wouldn't want the bad foods anymore. To make the biggest positive change you can for your health, all it takes is a little will power for a few weeks. There's just one thing—don't step on the weighing scale for the first two weeks. This is only because most people expect to lose weight on the second day, and when they don't, it dampens their spirit.

After about two to three weeks, your metabolism will become stable, and you will begin to feel like a new person. You will notice your clothes loosening up. Now, you can get on the weighing scale. You will see the results of your weight loss not only in the way your clothes fit, but also on the scale. You have slowly but surely started treading the right path.

The biggest hurdle for people is going through the initial withdrawal stage. The feelings and effects of your changes will be noticeable at first and might be hard to bear, but it is at this time you need to deal with it, knowing that when you do, your body will take on a new shape and look, and you will feel like a million bucks in just a few weeks. Making this small sacrifice for only a couple of weeks is one of the most impactful things you can do to be healthy, slim and full of energy for the rest of your life. It's a small price to pay for a lifetime of health.

Top Fat-Burning and Metabolism Booster Foods in the Great Indian Diet

1. Almonds: A study by the University of Toronto found that people who ate almonds with white bread didn't experience the same blood sugar surges as those who ate just a slice of bread. The higher the rise in blood sugar levels, the lower the fall will be. That dip leads to hunger, causing people to overeat. Moreover, blood sugar changes cause the body to make insulin, which can increase abdominal fat.

This weight loss food is replete with important nutrients like monounsaturated fats, vitamin E, folic acid, protein and dietary fibre. Almonds work best as a quick healthy snack when you are travelling or are at your office desk, or the moment when you want to hog something unhealthy. It also keeps your blood sugar steady.

2. Fruit: A majority of fruits, like apples, pears, oranges and watermelon, are high in fibre and water content, are full of antioxidants and are low in calories, making them ideal snacks to munch on to satisfy hunger pangs, eat as pre- and post-workout meals, and as a healthy dessert option. The fibre content in fruits keeps your cholesterol and blood sugar levels in check. Fibre helps give a feeling of satiety and prevents over-eating. When your body is healthy, your metabolism is high. Fruits like avocado contain healthy fats which help in the quick conversion of fats to energy without getting stored in the body. Tomatoes stimulate the production of an amino acid, carnitine, which is known to speed up the body's fat burning capacity.

3. Whole Grains and Beans: Excellent sources of fibre and protein and low in fat content, whole grains and beans help maintain your cholesterol, blood sugar and blood pressure levels. A lean body burns more calories than a body with a sluggish metabolism.

4. Vegetables: Similar to fruits, vegetables are high in fibre and antioxidants, are low in calories and on the glycemic index, and are therefore ideal for weight loss programmes. The antioxidants in them strengthen the body's immune system. A healthy body is endowed with a healthy metabolism. Green, leafy vegetables, like spinach, broccoli, kale, etc., are rich in iron which helps in improving the blood, oxygen and nutrient transporting capacity of the body and hence speeds up the metabolism. Vegetables like cabbage, cauliflower, carrot, cucumber and sweet potato can be consumed in the form of soups, unstrained juices, and stir-fried vegetables, satisfying our hunger without increasing our weight and aiding in the fat burning capacity of the body by keeping its metabolism at its peak.

5. Cinnamon: Cinnamon is a great weight loss ingredient. Just half a teaspoon of it each day can help control blood sugar and prevent post-meal insulin spikes that can trigger the body to store fat rather than burn it. This nutty flavoured spice is also known for its diabetes-fighting properties. Cinnamon can work wonders for your sweet tooth, while keeping you at a safe distance from fatty sugars and desserts. Not only that, it promotes effective blood circulation, which helps you get fitter faster. Add ground cinnamon as a replacement for sugar in cake dough or in your tea and coffee to get the most out of this wonderful spice every day.

6. Lentils: Lentils are the fastest and easiest foods to prepare, while also being one of the most popular ingredients in Indian kitchens. Dals can reduce your chances of a heart attack, stabilize sugar levels and help in weight loss. Lentils are a bona fide belly flattener. They are high in protein and soluble fibre, two nutrients that stabilize blood sugar levels. Eating these helps prevent insulin spikes that cause your body to create excess fat, especially in the abdominal area. This weight loss food is perfect for diabetic patients and also improves your iron and vitamin B levels. It is not only a comfort food but also a good source of protein for vegetarians.

7. Bananas: According to HMU expert Arnav Sarkar, bananas are part of a healthy diet, and should also be part of a fat loss diet. However, no food by itself can help one lose weight. One has to create a caloric deficit, that is burn more calories than are consumed in a day.

In most cases, a caloric deficit of 10 to 15 per cent works best, and a higher caloric deficit generally causes more muscle loss than fat loss. For starters, bananas offer healthy carbs that provide energy to be more active and feel great. It also has a level of potassium, which helps lower blood pressure. The fibre content of bananas helps control hunger much better for those who are trying to lose fat. It helps relieve constipation. Did you know that bananas have also been found to help students study better as a result of the vitamin B_6 in it?

Eating bananas has been found to reduce depression due to their tryptophan content. This fruit is also great for those afflicted by an emia as the iron content in it helps counter their condition. Breakfast is the best time to have bananas. You can chop them and add them to a bowl of milk with a few strawberries.

8. Coconut Oil: Coconut oil, with its medium chain fatty acids, aids in easy and quick digestion and detoxification thus reducing the load on the liver and helping in burning fats. Coconut oil is also known to kickstart slow functioning thyroid glands, thus ensuring a quicker metabolism.

9. Cabbage: This weight loss food is found in every continent, so you have no excuse to shy away from it. Cabbage is the ideal vegetable for those suffering from constipation, skin and eye disorders, ageing, stomach ulcers and Alzheimer's disease, among others. It is very low in calories and high in fibre. In addition, cabbage is extremely low on the glycemic index. This weight loss vegetable doesn't just help you lose weight. It is also a surprisingly excellent source of vitamin C, which some experts believe might reduce the risk of developing diabetes.

10. Eggs: Eggs are an excellent source of proteins which help us build muscles and get a lean physique. Protein puts the body at work. It needs to work harder and uses more energy to digest proteins. When you consume more proteins, you automatically reduce your carbohydrates. Extra carbohydrates consumed are converted into fat and stored in the body.

11. Coffee: The caffeine in coffee can raise your resting metabolic rate by about 15 per cent, and the effect can last up to four hours—which adds up to an extra 30–50 calories burned per day. Also, people who sip three to four cups of regular or decaffeinated coffee per day are 30 per cent less prone to developing type-2 diabetes.

12. Turmeric: This powerful extract of the turmeric root cleanses the liver and boosts metabolism. It is known to infuse the body with antioxidants and is also highly anti-inflammatory in nature.

13. Green Tea: Green tea contains substances called catechins and polyphenols. These two substances work in the body to force it to release stored fat.

14. Lemons: This highly alkaline vegetable balances the pH level in the body, making it more alkaline, which is the best condition for fat loss to take place. Research has also shown that diseases usually thrive and breathe in acidic conditions. It's an excellent habit to keep the body alkaline by incorporating lemons into your diet. Lemons are full of vitamin C, and thereby also help build immunity.

15. Capsaicin: One ingredient that nutritionists say helps people lose weight is capsaicin. It is an active compound found in chilli and cayenne peppers.

It causes an increase in the metabolic rate. When this happens, your body burns calories. This, in turn, forces your body to burn fat. So, if you can stand to eat something spicy, you may want to try some chilli and cayenne peppers.

The Great Indian Diet Plan

What Is Your Weight?

Most of us are obsessed by how much we weigh. It has become a number that is discussed as much as politics, sports, and the weather. In many cases, people are ashamed to talk about their weight or even stand on weighing scales. There are also several people who are obsessed with weighing themselves. Some do it every day, some after every meal, and some every two hours. Each time you step on those scales it is like a test. What few people remember is that body weight can fluctuate. Everybody's weight goes up and down, even of fit and slim people. Your weight can fluctuate by as much as four to five kilos due to environmental factors, water retention, and even atmospheric pressure changes. In short, there is no point being obsessed with the weighing scale. You will know whether you are fat or slim by how you look or feel. When you fit into your clothes better, and lose inches, it means you have lost fat and that's all that matters. Being slim, however, is not a marker of good health. You might be at your ideal weight on the scale and yet your arteries might be clogged. The weighing scale is the smallest and most negligible part of your journey to get fit and healthy. Don't let it become an obstacle.

The Weighing Scale

The oldest evidence for the existence of weighing scales dates to 2400 to 1800 BCE in the Indus Valley Civilization. In Egypt, scales can be traced to around 1878 BCE. In the medieval times, Egyptian merchants used an established system of weight measurement to catalogue gold shipments or gold mine yields. Henceforth, weighing scales were used by traders to weigh spices, cotton, and so on. In modern times, weighing scales began to be used by doctors to determine if a patient was underweight or overweight. Today even a 100 gram to 300 gram shift in the scale can worry, frustrate, and make us angry, or push us to lose kilos.

I strongly feel that we should focus on fat loss and not weight loss. (We have spoken about fat loss in detail in Chapter Seven.) On a scale, you could be losing weight and that could be anything but fat. It could be weight due to water, or healthy lean mass because of poor nutrition.

Don't let the scale reading play on your mind and demotivate you. Instead, shift your focus from the scale to being consistent with your food, exercise, sleep and emotional health, and fat loss will surely follow.

Learn to Balance Your Diet

For me, it is simple. At home and outside, we eat good food, and we also eat junk once in a while. What balances it all is discipline. My husband, Raj, loves food, and there's nothing wrong with that. I love great food too, but we have learnt to find a balance. I have a sweet tooth and love eating Indian desserts. Sunday is our 'cheat day', and the Kundra family eats pretty much anything. We all enjoy food and I love trying out different cuisines. I rarely eat junk food and usually ask myself a few questions before consuming anything. Will the food I'm going to eat provide me with nutrition? Or is it just going to line my intestines and slow down my digestive process? I would rather have a rasmalai which is cottage cheese in milk, even though it has sugar, rather than a gulab jamun which is deep fried. Sometimes, I have a piece of chikki when I feel I really need to battle a sweet craving and it usually does the trick.

My husband's concept of desserts, however, is completely different. In the UK, when they serve you a slice of cake, it is almost a quarter of a kilo. So when I give him a thin slice he wants more. He says, 'I want a real piece, not a slice to taste.' So we enjoy our foods and desserts but we also follow a certain discipline that uses moderation and compensation as the main tools. There are times when you go out or if you are travelling, and you see a really well-made tiramisu. If you want to have it, just have it, don't think twice about it. Never eat your food with guilt. It's not only about the food you eat. It's a lot to do with how you eat it. Later in this book, we will talk about the whole mind–body connection and the stress–guilt impact on your body and weight.

I see a lot of Indians cutting back on oil completely in an attempt to lose weight. That's wrong. Good oils are required by the human body and it's important that it be part of your diet. As we have discussed, India has some of the healthiest oils in the world and we should eventually return to using those local oils.

All That Fizz

Aerated drinks are like a slow poison for our bodies. Imagine the harm they can inflict on children if they are so unhealthy for adults. What about diet sodas? Aren't they sugar-free and healthy? Diet sodas lead to a fat build up around the liver and skeletal muscles. They can contribute towards insulin resistance and increase cholesterol in your body. When the liver encounters excess glucose, it is converted to body fat.

A non-profit centre for science, in a public interest petition told the US agency, Food and Drug Administration (FDA), to ban the artificial brown colouring used in certain aerated beverages. There are two contaminants in the colouring—2-methylimidazole and 4-methylimidazole—which have been found to cause cancer in animals. Just 16 micrograms per person per day of 4-methylimidazole is enough to pose a cancer threat and most popular brown aerated beverages, diet and regular, contain 200 micrograms in every 20 ounce bottle. Brown aerated beverages contain phosphates or phosphoric acid, a weak acid that gives these beverages their tangy flavour and shelf life. Several dairy and meat products have these chemicals too, so please check the labels carefully. Too much phosphoric acid leads to heart and kidney problems, muscle loss, osteoporosis and accelerates aging. There is so a lot of research that proves how dangerous aerated drinks are, and even worse is when these are used as mixers with alcohol, forming a lethal concoction that causes harm to vital organs and the body.

Did you know that almost all aerated drinks contain dangerous ingredients, many of which are carcinogenic and many of them work together to rob the body of calcium, magnesium and other important trace minerals? They contain everything from aspartame to a host of other artificial sweeteners, to Ace-K, saccharin, sodium cyclamate, (sucralose) E955, maltodextrin, high-fructose corn syrup, phosphorus, caramel color, and other chemicals that are disastrous to the health of adults and children. We cannot stress enough the importance of banning sodas for your children. There is absolutely no excuse. There is enough evidence that links the addictive effect of aerated drinks to that of cocaine and heroin and it hampers your child's growth, promotes hormonal imbalance, weakens and softens bones and teeth.

In cancer research, we learn that consuming a single can of an aerated drink brings down the immunity by almost 70 per cent and this effect lasts for over four hours. By now we all know what can happen when we have weak immunity and how important it is to avoid things that weaken this intelligent system that is designed to protect us, heal and cure us.

We love referring to this link (http://www. seattleorganicrestaurants.com/vegan-whole-food/Pepsi-Coca-Cola-harmful-ingredients.php) that lays out so well, what happens in our bodies when we consume these toxic concoctions.

The first 10 minutes: Within ten minutes of drinking sodas, ten teaspoons of sugar hit your system (100 per cent more than the recommended daily sugar intake) and phosphoric acid cuts the overwhelming sweetness and that's the only reason that you won't throw up.

Within 20 minutes: Your body will experience an insulin burst as your blood sugar spikes while your liver turns massive amount of sugar into fat.

Within 40 minutes: Your body has absorbed caffeine so your blood pressure goes up and your liver dumps more sugar into your bloodstream.

Within 45 minutes: Your body releases more dopamine (dopamine stimulates the pleasure centres of the brain)—the same reaction that addicts have to drugs like heroin.

After 60 minutes: Phosphoric acid binds magnesium, zinc and calcium in your lower intestine and high levels of artificial sweeteners (like aspartame) or sugar increases excretion of calcium via urine. The caffeine will also come to play by dehydrating your body and you will lose a lot of water by going to bathroom. Phosphoric acid and caffeine also deplete your body from the bonded magnesium, zinc and calcium as well as sodium, electrolyte and water that were headed to your bones. After losing the valuable nutrients in your body that could have been used for hydrating or building stronger bones and teeth, you get a sugar rush before your system crashes.

I remember I was in Goa when a client called and explained how she was diagnosed with fibroids and cysts in her breasts and ovary. We went over her lifestyle and food habits, and what stood out was her consumption of two cans of an aerated drink per day with her meals. The only advice she got from me was to replace that with lemon water, and we added a few sprigs of mint to give it flavour. She was exercising regularly and sleeping well. Two months later she repeated her tests and everything was normal. Hard to believe, but it's true.

Patients suffering from PCOD (poly-cystic ovarian disease), fibroids, cysts, gastric disorders, high levels of cholesterol and triglycerides, and diabetes, experience significant improvement in their health on quitting sodas. Patients diagnosed as pre-diabetic were completely healed when they stopped consuming these beverages. The best part was how cutting out these drinks allowed for a natural and healthy balance of hormones in women, leading to better and less painful menstrual cycles, a seamless menopause, reduction in migraines and headaches, and even improvement in cases of depression. When it came to weight loss, cutting out these drinks rapidly decreased abdominal fat and cellulite in most people.

Aerated drinks rob the bones and cells of nutrition, making them weak and leading to teeth, bone, spinal, knee, and immunity disorders. There are so many healthy options in the great Indian diet. We suggest the good old soda or water with some fresh lemon, sweetened with jaggery or pure honey. This combination is a powerfully refreshing health drink that can eventually replace the sugar- and chemical-filled evil concoctions.

It is important that adults and children know that a created beverages are designed to get you addicted and that's the reason why consumers find it so difficult to give them up. The worst combination is of junk food and aerated drinks, which robs your cells of nutrition, spikes your insulin levels, makes you hungry and crave salt. They deposit a large amount of toxins in your system, which puts your liver in overdrive to clean, not to mention the ugly cellulite that hangs on to your midriff and sides, all due to the high-fructose corn syrup which is worse than white sugar. It destroys immunity, which is your only line of defence when it comes to protecting you from disease.

We have a common piece of advice for parents who wish to improve their children's nutrition, as they feel their child is too tired to focus in class and participate in sports. It is, 'Don't let your kids have aerated drinks; offer them healthy substitutes instead.' The parents are surprised when the child starts to feel active, energetic and shows drastic improvement in activities at school, when they had thought the child needed supplements and medication. The truth is that some of the most complex problems are solved with simple solutions, and we have to believe that something as small and insignificant as a can of aerated drink can mess up the human body and brain. When these things happen and kids start to get affected, parents blame the school, teachers, food, too much homework and other stuff. The solution could just be in the kind of junk they feed their kids.

Why You May Not Be Losing Weight

Are you doing all the right things and still finding it difficult to shed those pounds? Have a look at this list below. We call them 'derailment factors' that can sabotage your weight loss, resulting in frustration and low motivation levels.

1. Skipping your breakfast or having a skimpy breakfast
2. Thyroid imbalance
3. High intake of G.I. foods (glycemic index), such as white sugar, white flour, baked and processed goods
4. Consuming aerated drinks
5. Your workout has gotten monotonous and your body is used to the pace. Mix it up with interval or high intensity training
6. You are eating 'low fat' foods. Take a peek at the label and you will find it loaded with sugar
7. The frequency of eating out at restaurants is high
8. You are not keeping a gap of two to three hours between supper and bed-time
9. Excessive consumption of alcohol
10. Smoking
11. More than three hours' gap between meals
12. Acidity and bloating. You can make your system alkaline by increasing the amounts of fruits, vegetable and lemon in your food plan
13. Following fad diets discussed in social circles. Everyone has a different body type and what works for one may in fact harm you
14. Constipation. Increase your consumption of raw vegetables, water, fruits and fibre-rich carbohydrates
15. Liver problems

16. You eat too fast and don't chew your food properly
17. Check your stress levels. This should actually be at the top of the list

Reflect on this list. Sometimes, just changing a few of these things or even just one can start getting you amazing results.

The Great Indian Diet

This book will take you through a journey of great Indian foods and at the end of it all, you will be equipped to build your own food plan for yourself or your family. It's really simple when you are clearly aware of your goal. You couple that with knowledge, a dose of discipline, and the right attitude to achieve the body and health you really want. Whenever you search the internet for a diet plan, you will come across plans that are suited for Western culture. If you are an Indian and have spent most part of your life in India munching on a wide variety of Indian foods, it would be difficult to follow an American diet plan. You will be longing to find an Indian diet plan that will help you reduce weight so that you can eat what you have been eating so far and yet lose weight. The following is an Indian weight loss diet chart that you need to follow to shed the extra kilos easily.

Best Vegetarian Diet for Weight Loss

As said earlier, the calorie requirement of every person is different and some people prefer vegetarian food

The 1,200 Calorie Vegetarian Indian Diet Plan

By following this menu guide, you will be able to restrict your food consumption to just 1,200 to 1,300 calories a day. You will feel lighter after a couple of weeks of following this weight loss diet menu.

The vegetarian diet menu is as follows:

Early Morning (7 a.m.)
- A glass of lukewarm water with lemon (0 calories)
- A cup of tea with skimmed milk, no sugar and two biscuits (90 calories)

Breakfast (8 a.m.)
- 2 wheat rotis or chapatis + ½ cup paneer gravy, though tofu is better (330 calories).

Or
- A plate of brown bread upma and a cup of skimmed milk (300 calories)

Mid-morning Snack (10:30 a.m.)
- A banana or 20 grapes or ½ cup melon (50 calories)

Lunch (1 p.m.)
- 1 cup brown rice (200 grams) + ½ cup mixed vegetables + one small bowl of raita + 1 bowl vegetable salad (345 calories)

Evening (4 p.m.)
- Buttermilk 1 glass or 1 cup (35 calories)

Dinner (8 p.m.)
- 2 chapatis or rotis + 1 bowl of vegetable soup + 1 bowl of salad (370 calories)

The total calories you will consume in this vegetarian diet are about 1,220 calories.

The 1,200 Calorie Non-Vegetarian Indian Diet Plan Menu

If you are a non-vegetarian and do not like the idea of eating a lot of vegetables to lose weight, there is no need to worry. You can lose a considerable amount of weight by including non-vegetarian dishes in your daily menu. The following is a non-vegetarian Indian diet plan for weight loss.

Early Morning (7 a.m.)
- A glass of lukewarm water with lemon (0 calories)
- A cup of tea with skimmed milk, no sugar and two biscuits (90 calories)

Breakfast (8 a.m.)
- 2 slices of brown bread + 2 hardboiled eggs (290 calories)

Or
- 1 slice of brown bread + 2 scrambled eggs + 1 cup skimmed milk without sugar (310 calories)

Mid-morning Snack (10:30 a.m.)
- A banana or 20 grapes or ½ cup melon or a fistful of almonds or walnuts (50 calories)

Lunch (1 p.m.)
- 1 cup brown rice (200 grams) + ½ cup mixed vegetables + 100 grams of chicken (boiled or stir-fried in olive oil) + 1 bowl of vegetable salad (360 calories)

Evening (4 p.m.)
- Buttermilk 1 glass or 1 cup (35 calories)

Dinner (8 p.m.)
1 chapati or roti + ½ cup of lentils (dal) + 50 grams of fish (rich in omega-3 fatty acids) + 1 bowl of raita (380 calories)

The total number of calories you will consume in a day by following this non-vegetarian diet menu is 1,225 calories.

while others prefer non-vegetarian food. Whatever be the type of food you have, there should be some caloric deficit so that the body starts using its stored fat. The minimum daily energy requirement for an adult human being is 1,200 to 1,800 calories. Hence, your diet should be restricted within 1,800 calories. Make sure that you divide the 1,800 calories into three meals per day and healthy snacks twice daily to achieve the best possible result within a short period of time. Here is a guideline for creating the best vegetarian diet for weight loss. Based on this, you can create your own diet plan as the food choices of each person may vary and the items available to you may be different from those mentioned here.

Following this diet plan, you will be able to lose weight by eating all your favourite foods. You will not need to do rigorous workouts; mild exercises are enough. If you are looking to lose weight within a short span of time, then the 1,200 calorie diet plan will help you shed the extra kilos by making a little bit of an adjustment to your lifestyle and diet.

We strongly recommend that you be aware of foods that have good and bad, high and low calories and balance your daily food plan accordingly.

The reason for sharing these sample plans is that you understand how to create a food plan structure based on your goals, whether it is weight loss, healing, prevention, or just living healthy and eating well. The rest of this book will help you select the foods you need and formulate your own food plan.

* * *

I want so share a story with a before and after picture of a lovely lady, who lives in Hyderabad and used a simple Indian diet to produce these fantastic results in her weight, health and lifestyle.

Aarti's Story

I weighed 122 kilos when I was thirty-eight years of age. This is how I looked like then and this is how I look now.

Today I weigh 100 kilos after seven months under Luke's guidance.

I live in a joint family. My husband is a prosthodontist by profession. I am a teacher and teach kindergarten at a school owned by my mother. I love cooking, listening to music and travelling. Initially I religiously followed Luke's plan but later, as I grew confident and comfortable with the food I was eating, I started alternating with other healthy options which I would eat only after asking Luke.

My day started with lime water and cinnamon followed by breakfast, which was usually idli, oats or a vegetable sandwich.

I started eating every two hours. The foods I inculcated in my diet included fruits, almonds, walnuts, buttermilk and green tea. I prefer to eat vegetables rather than juicing them, so I ate raw vegetables instead. I ate an apple or a cucumber whenever I felt hungry. My lunch would be chapati and vegetables with curd and dal. I usually had salad and some protein or vegetables, and ended with green tea and fresh lemon.

What I think worked for me is the simplicity of the food plan, the fact that I could enjoy Indian foods, and the discipline in eating habits. Eating right at the right time made a huge difference. I am so grateful to Luke for his patience, continuous motivation and dedication. His willingness to help and the confidence he shows in you makes you believe that it's not difficult to lose weight at all.

The only exercise I did was walking. I started with a twenty-minute walk every evening and slowly increased it to forty minutes. To be honest, I had never thought I would be able to lose weight. Now I am more energetic, healthy, my skin looks great, and I feel positive.

Shilpa's Diet Plan

I used the great Indian diet to maintain the body and health I have today. It helped me prepare for a great pregnancy and rapidly lose all the weight I gained during that time. No matter what diet you choose, you should be aware of your life and the way you live. Yes, it's true that height, weight and your genes do play a role, but too many people focus on just that. There is so much more that we need to be aware of, that contributes towards a healthy body and weight.

Wake up with lemon water and a cup of green tea with pure honey.

Breakfast:
- Four grain mix (jowar, bajra, nachni, wheat) or whole wheat toast with paneer bhurji or tofu

Or
- Broken wheat upma or daliya and low fat milk

Or
- Two idlis with half a cup sambhar and half a cup low fat milk with green tea

Mid-morning Snack:
- Papaya with a dash of lemon or a low fat yogurt with mixed fruits

Lunch:
- Red or brown rice (small bowl)

Or
- Two moong dal chilla

Or
- Two rotis (mixed grains) with vegetables plus low fat yoghurt and dal

(You can have a clear soup, salad or raw carrots before lunch.)

Evening snack:
- Green tea or half a cup oats cooked in water

Or
- Fruit and nuts

Or
- A small bowl of air-popped popcorn or makhanas with a little ghee and pepper

Dinner:
- A thin soup plus roti and vegtables

Or
- Oats upma with vegetable curry

(If you have 10 kilos to lose, you must alternate every second day with a low carb, no carb diet.)
- Lemon water

Non-vegetarians can replace paneer with eggs (two whites and one yolk) and at night, three egg whites with one yolk, with onions, chilli, parsley and coriander or steamed fish or chicken at night with a clear soup. A raw carrot is a must with every meal.

As dessert, you can have a piece of jaggery three times a week after lunch or a peanut-based jaggery chikki or homemade sesame (til) ladoos.

Most importantly, dinner should be had as early as possible, preferably before 8 p.m.

Also, I would advise women over thirty-five to have a multi-vitamin and calcium tablet post-lunch.

My binge day is Sunday, but up to 6 p.m., and I never regret what I eat. Eating with guilt or fear is worse for your body as cortisol levels are elevated when the body is stressed and cortisol tells your body to store fat.

Shilpa's Post-Pregnancy Diet

7:30 a.m. 15 ml aloe vera juice plus ten tulsi leaves, jaggery and ginger

7:45 a.m. Warm water (two glasses)

8 a.m. Oats in water with a dash of milk, or museli in skimmed milk, or two whole eggs with whole wheat toast plus five almonds soaked overnight

9 a.m. Tea with milk and brown sugar

11 a.m. Papaya or musk melon, apple or strawberry, orange and five tablespoons yogurt smoothie

1 p.m. Lunch of brown rice with a teaspoon of ghee (one bowl) + vegetable + chicken or fish grilled. Or Beans + one raw carrot + one glass chaas (salted with roasted jeera) + one raw carrot

Dessert – a piece of peanut or jaggery chikki or dudhi halwa made with raisins and dates (twice a week until I lost 10 kilos)

3:30 p.m. Eight to ten roasted makhanas, or five walnuts and raisins, or crackers with low fat hummus or avacado dip, or two scrambled eggs

7:30 p.m. For dinner, mixed vegetable soup (pumpkin, tomato, greens), or clear chicken soup + salad (sprouts, tomato, apple, beetroot, lettuce, chaat masala). Until I lost the first 10 kilos, I had just soup and moong dal pancakes for dinner

Main course – Moong dal chillas with paneer, or grilled stir-fried chicken with veggies, or steamed braised fish with beans or broccoli and mushroom + one raw carrot.

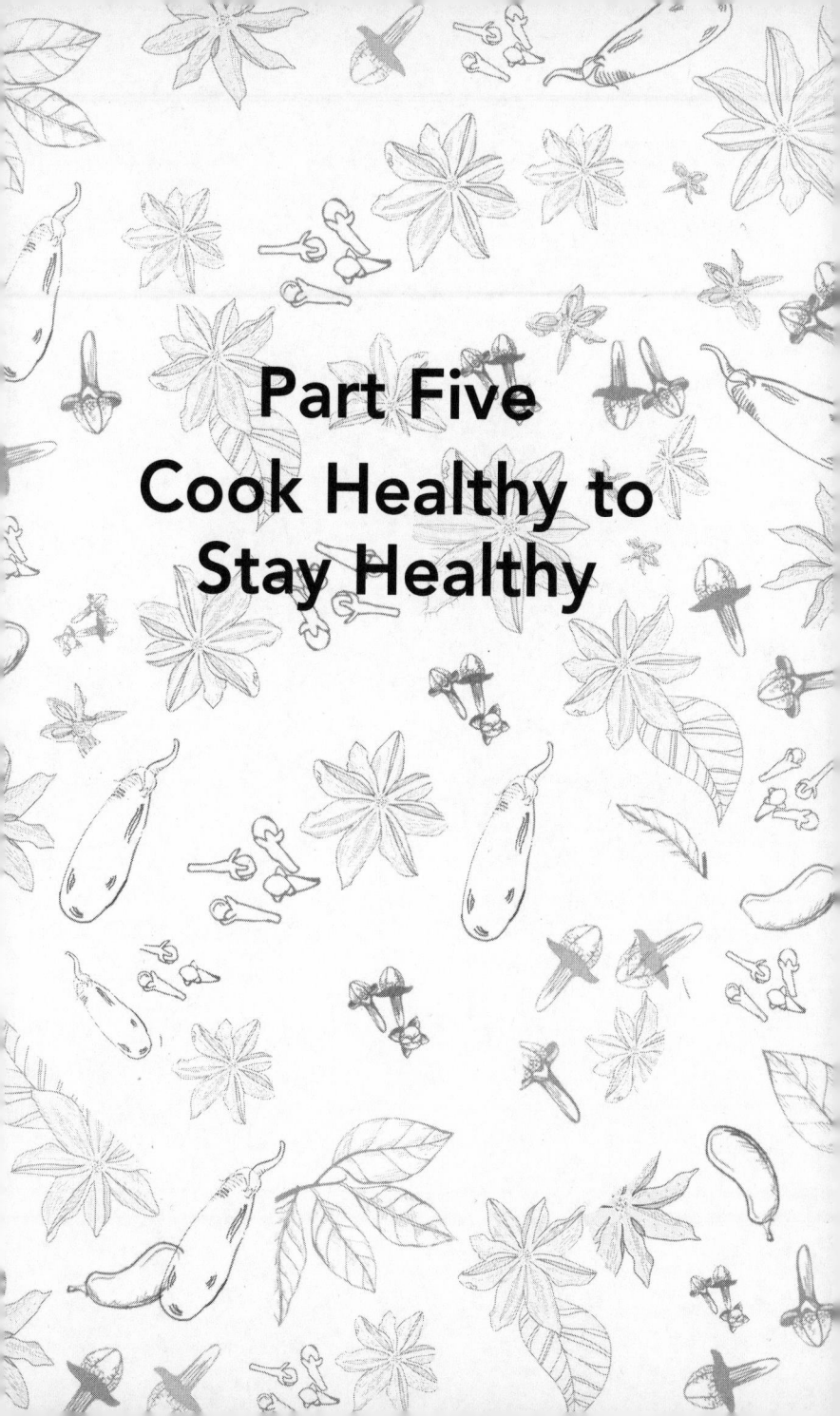

Part Five
Cook Healthy to Stay Healthy

Recipes for the Great Indian Diet

In this chapter, we will share some of our favorite recipes and super-healthy juices with you to help you lose weight and enhance your health.

Say Hello to Salads

- **Beetroot Salad**

   Beetroots: 2
   Mustard seeds: ¼ tsp
   Coconut oil: 1 tsp
   Curry leaves: 4 to 5
   Heeng: A pinch
   Salt and pepper to taste

Boil and cut the beetroot into cubes. Heat oil in a pan, add the mustard seeds and curry leaves, heeng and beetroot. Add grated coconut and coriander leaves (optional). Can be served hot or cold.

- **French Bean and Peanut Salad**

  French beans: 500 grams
  Coconut oil: 1 tsp
  Garlic: 4 cloves, finely chopped
  Peanuts: 4 to 5, toasted and crushed
  Salt and pepper to taste

De-string and cut the beans one into two. Heat oil in a pan, add garlic and fry till golden brown. Add the peanuts and beans. Add salt and pepper to taste. Can be served hot or cold.

- **Bean Salad**

  Beans or lentils: 2 cups, cooked
  Onion: 1 chopped
  Tomato: 1 chopped
  Coriander: A handful, chopped
  Cumin: 1 tsp
  Salt and chaat masala to taste
  Chilli powder: ½ tsp (optional)

It can be made with all kinds of beans, or by mixing two types of lentils too.

Boil the beans or lentils, with chopped onion, tomato, ginger, coriander, jeera, salt and chilli (optional).

After they are cooked, strain the water but don't throw it away.

Sprinkle the chaat masala and eat with low fat yogurt and roasted moong papad.

The water can be had as a plain soup or you can add carrots and a few grains of brown rice and squeeze a bit of lime to make it a full meal.

- **Paneer**

  > Paneer: 500 grams
  > Lettuce/long beans/parboiled spinach: 250 grams
  > Cumin powder: 1 tsp
  > Salt and pepper to taste
  > Dressing:
  > Orange juice: 2 tbsp
  > Olive oil: 1 tbsp
  > Lemon: ½
  > Yellow mustard mix: ¼ tsp

Roast paneer in a non-stick pan without oil, lightly browning both the sides. Add salt, pepper and jeera powder, chilli powder is optional.

Mix in lettuce leaves, long beans or parboiled spinach.

For the dressing, take two spoons of orange juice, olive oil, a dash of lemon, a quarter spoon of yellow mustard mix, and add to the above.

This can be combined with sautéed mushrooms or carrots, and instead of paneer you can use boiled eggs too.

This recipe can create a complete and filling dinner for working women who don't have time to cook elaborate meals.

Veggies Show the Way

- **Rice Noodles with Vegetable or Seviyan**

  > Rice noodles or gluten-free noodles
  > Spring onions
  > Zucchini: 1
  > Capsicum: 1

Garlic: A few cloves
Olive oil
Salt and pepper to taste

Mix the above ingredients with the noodles, but without soya.

- **Rawa Dhokla**

    Idli rawa: 1 glass
    Slim Yogurt: ½ cup
    Water: 1 glass
    Vegetable oil: 1 tsp
    Fruit salt: ½ tsp
    Rock salt: ½ tsp
    Tempering:
    Ghee/vegetable oil: 1 tsp
    Mustard seeds: ¼ tsp
    Haldi: ¼ tsp
    Red chillies powder: ¼ tsp
    Curry leaves: 4
    Heeng: ¼ tsp

Mix all the ingredients, with the exception of the tempering ingredients, and keep aside for thirty minutes to ferment. Spread half teaspoon oil on to the thali. Add the batter. Steam for twelve to fifteen minutes.

Heat ghee or oil in a pan. Add the mustard seeds, heeng, curry leaves, haldi and chilly powder.

Once the dhokla is ready. Cut diagonally and add the tempering on top.

Optional: Add freshly grated coconut and coriander leaves.

- **Stir-Fried Mushrooms**

  > Vegetable oil: 1 tsp
  > Onion: ½ or Spring onions: 3
  > Ginger: 1 inch
  > Vinegar: 1 tsp
  > White button mushrooms: 8
  > Capsicum: 1
  > Green Chilly (de-seeded): 1
  > Salt and pepper to taste

Heat the oil. Stir-fry the onions, ginger, capsicum and green chilly. Add mushrooms, vinegar, salt and pepper to taste.

Non-Vegetarian Delicacies

- **Grilled Fish**

  > Fish fillets of your choice: 4
  > Coriander or pudina paste: ½ bowl
  > Ginger: 1 tsp
  > Garlic: 1 tsp
  > Lemon Juice: 1 tsp
  > Chilli powder: ½ tsp
  > Turmeric: ½ tsp
  > Mustard or coconut oil: ½ tsp

Marinate in mint or coriander paste, garlic, ginger, lemon juice, chilli powder, turmeric, salt and mustard or coconut oil. Crush and apply on the fish before grilling for seven to ten minutes. You can steam or microwave for twelve to fifteen minutes, depending on how you like it.

- **Grilled chicken**

  > Boneless chicken pieces: ½ kg
  > Hung or low fat curd: 2 tsp
  > Jeera: 1 tsp
  > Coriander powder: 1 tsp
  > Ginger paste: 1 tsp
  > Turmeric: ½ tsp
  > Garam masala (optional): ½ tsp
  > Chilli powder (optional): 1 tsp
  > Pepper: ½ tsp
  > Lemon juice: 1 tsp
  > Salt to taste
  > Ghee: 1 tsp

Marinate chicken in hung or low fat curd, jeera, coriander, ginger, turmeric, garam masala (optional), chilli (optional), pepper, lemon juice, salt, and olive oil that keeps it moist. Grill or microwave for fifteen minutes and enjoy.

- **Stir-fried mushroom (with chicken optional)**

  > Boneless Chicken: 250 gm
  > Onion finely chopped: 1
  > Ghee: 1 tsp
  > Ginger garlic paste: 1 ½ tsp
  > Vinegar: ½ tsp
  > Salt to taste
  > Capsicum finely chopped: 2
  > Mushroom finely chopped: 500 gm

Heat ghee in a non-stick pan. Add garlic, onion followed by chicken marinated in ginger-garlic paste, vinegar and salt. Saute for two to three minutes then add capsicums and mushrooms. Your stir fry mushroom will be ready in ten minutes. Serve with brown rice. It can be made with prawns or fish too.

Indian Recipes for Weight Loss

Let's now learn how to make some of the tastiest Indian recipes that will also help you lose weight.

1. Ragi

Ragi is a popular annual plant that is loaded with healthy nutrients. It is a good source of iron, protein, calcium and other minerals. It is also rich in fibre and aids in weight loss as it contains negligible saturated fats. It will help control diabetes, cholesterol and blood pressure, and is also known to help in digestion. The following are some ragi recipes that will help you lose weight.

a) Ragi Shake

You must have had mango shake, banana shake and chocolate shake. But have you ever tried ragi shake? Ragi shake is an Indian version of an energy drink popular in South India. It keeps you fresh and active throughout the day.

Ingredients
- Ragi flour: 1 cup
- Skimmed milk: ½ cup
- Water: 2 cups
- Jaggery, powdered: 2 tbsp
- Cardamom powder: 1½ tsp

Take a bowl and add the ragi flour. Pour the water and stir it into a smooth paste so that no lumps are formed. Now take a pan and heat the skimmed milk till it comes to a boil. Add the ragi paste, cardamom powder and keep on stirring it. Add the jaggery powder and cook for four to five minutes on a low flame. Keep on stirring continuously to avoid the lumps from forming. Cool it before you enjoy your healthy ragi shake.

b) **Upma Made with Ragi**

Upma is a popular South Indian breakfast and if it is made with ragi, the health benefits get multiplied. It is also filling and will keep you away from nibbling on junk food during the course of the day.

Ingredients
- Ragi flour: 2 cups
- Mustard seeds: ½ tsp
- Ghee: 1 ½ tsp
- Black gram: ½ tsp
- Bengal gram: ½ tsp
- Onion, finely chopped: 2
- Tomato, finely chopped: 1
- Green chillies, finely chopped: 3
- Coriander leaves, finely chopped: 1 tbsp
- Curry leaves: 8 to 10
- Water: 4 cups
- Haldi: ½ tsp
- Lemon juice: 2 tsp

Take a saucepan and heat the ghee. Add the ragi flour and sauté it for two to three minutes. Keep aside. Take another pan and add a little ghee followed by mustard seeds. After you hear the crackling sound, add the Bengal gram followed by the black gram. Sauté them for a few minutes and then add onions and the curry leaves. Cook for another couple of minutes. To this add the tomatoes and cook for a minute. Add salt to taste and pour four cups of water. Let it boil. Then add the ragi and stir well for a couple of minutes. Now cover with a lid and cook for about five minutes on a low flame. Garnish with chopped coriander, pour lemon juice on it, and serve hot.

2. Oats

Super-rich in fibre, and also a great protein source, including oats in your diet is beneficial for weight loss, diabetes, controlling and reducing cholesterol, and cleaning the colon. It keeps you feeling full for a longer period of time, hence preventing you from snacking on unwanted calories. Oats makes for a great breakfast and also a powerful pre-workout meal.

a) Tangy Oats with Lemon
- Oats: 1cup
- Lemon juice: 1 ½ tbsp
- Water: 2 cups
- Haldi: ½ tsp
- Salt as per taste

For tempering
- Ghee: 2 tbsp
- Cumin seeds: ½ tsp
- Green chillies: 4 (slit)
- Peanuts: 1½ tbsp

- Black gram: 1½ tsp
- Bengal gram: 1 tbsp
- Coriander leaves: about a handful, washed and cut
- A pinch of asafoetida

Take a non-stick pan and heat it. Once it is hot, roast the oats for about two to three minutes on a low flame and keep aside. Now take another plan, add ghee and when it is hot add the tempering ingredients. Stir for a couple of minutes. To this add coriander, green chillies and turmeric followed by the peanuts. When the peanuts are light brown, add the water and bring it to a boil. To this add the oats and cook for about three to four minutes till it is done. Sprinkle lemon juice and serve hot.

b) Idli Made of Oats

When we are confused about what to eat for breakfast, both of us often go for the good old idli. This one made with oats tastes good, and is rich in fibre to boost your health. Since it requires very little oil to cook, it is an ideal weight loss recipe. You can also have it for lunch if you like.

- Oats: 2 cups
- Yoghurt: 1 cup
- Wheat rava: 1 cup
- Finely chopped mixed vegetables of your choice: 1½ cups
- Water: 2 cups
- Coriander leaves, finely chopped: 2 tbsp
- One sachet of Eno

For tempering
- Ghee: 1 tbsp
- Black gram: 1 tbsp
- Bengal gram: 1 tbsp
- Mustard: 1 tbsp
- Finely chopped green chillies: 1 tbsp
- Curry leaves: About 8-10

Take a non-stick pan and heat it. Once it is hot, roast the oats for about two to three minutes on a low flame and keep it aside. Once it cools down, make it into a powder in a blender. Now add ghee to a pan. When the ghee is hot, add the tempering ingredients and stir for a couple of minutes. Now add the vegetables and coriander leaves and cook for about three minutes. Add the rava and saute on a low flame for another couple of minutes. Place this mixture in a big bowl and add the blended oats, salt to taste, water, and curd. Mix it well to turn it into idli batter. Now add the Eno just before you want to make your delicious oats idlis. Once the idli plates are greased with a few drops of ghee, pour the batter and cook for fifteen to twenty minutes. Serve it hot with coconut or coriander chutney.

c) The Great Indian Oat Bowl
This is a great breakfast for kids as well as adults, and a great weight loss preparation too.
- Oats: 3-5 tbsp
- Milk/water
- Almonds (crushed): 5
- Flaxseed powder, freshly ground: 1 tbsp
- Pumpkin seeds: 1 tbsp

- Sunflower seeds: 1 tbsp
- A dash of cinnamon

Cook the oats in water and milk. Add all the nuts and seeds to it when it is nearly cooked, or you can even add when fully cooked. Sweeten the preparation with jaggery or pure honey. You can also add chopped dates, a teaspoon of black raisins, and pieces of fresh fruit like banana.

3. Tomatoes

Rich in lycopene, a phytochemical found in red vegetables, tomatoes have anti-inflammatory and antioxidant properties. You can easily include tomatoes in your diet with soups, which will reduce your appetite and thereby help in weight loss.

a) Masala Tomato Soup
- Tomatoes: 2
- Tomato puree: 2 tbsp
- Potatoes: 2
- Carrots: 2
- Onions: 2
- Water: 500 ml
- Vegetable stock: 500 ml
- Chilli powder: ½ tsp
- Salt to taste

Chop the onions, carrots and potatoes, and place in a pan along with the water and vegetable stock. Let it come to a boil. Then add the tomatoes, tomato puree, salt and chilli powder and allow it to simmer for a half an hour, while you stir it to prevent it from sticking to the bottom of the pan. If you need to, add more water. When it is done, allow it to cool and then whisk in a blender until it achieves the consistency of soup. Heat the soup before serving.

b) **Tomato Soup with Tulsi**
   - Tomatoes: 10
   - Tomato puree: 4 tbsp
   - Potato: 2 large
   - Onions: 2
   - Garlic: 6 to 7 cloves
   - Ginger: 1 inch piece
   - Ghee: 2 tbsp
   - Tulsi: 8 to 10 leaves
   - Salt to taste
   - Pepper to taste
   - Chilli flakes: ½ tsp

Heat the ghee in a saucepan and sauté the onions and garlic. Once they are soft, add the potatoes and fry for a minute. Pour in half a litre of water and let it come to a boil. Check the potatoes. When they are half-done, add the tomatoes and the puree. Allow them to cook on a slow flame until everything is well-done. Just prior to turning off the heat, add the chopped tulsi, salt and pepper. Serve the soup hot.

Healthy Vegetable Juices for Weight Loss

There is no doubt that consuming fresh vegetables and fruits will help you stay healthy and fit. These foods are considered excellent replacements for your daily meals. Juicing the vegetables is a good way to shed excess fat. It is one of the easiest and effective ways to lose excess body weight and is also loaded with a lot of nutrients. Vegetable juices will cleanse your body, help in weight loss as well as boost your metabolism. It has been found that drinking a glass of fresh vegetable juice every day will help lose weight quickly as juice gets easily absorbed by the body than actually eating the vegetables.

The following are some of the vegetable juices that you can consume for effective weight loss.

1.   Carrot Juice

Carrot juice is rich in dietary fibre and is also very good for improving eyesight. It will help promote higher levels of testosterone and reduce body fat. Carrot juices will also improve the body's self-defence mechanism. Drinking a glass of carrot juice every day after a gym session will help keep your stomach full till mealtime.

2.   Beetroot Juice

Another important vegetable juice that will aid weight loss and should be part of any weight loss diet is beetroot juice. It is full of nutrients and contains no cholesterol or fat. It will help you burn more calories while exercising and will also give you the strength and stamina for rigorous workouts. Beetroot juice has high fibre content and nutrients that will make you feel full all day long. Drinking a glass of beetroot juice for breakfast every morning will help provide you with the necessary soluble and insoluble dietary fibre as well as improve bowel movements.

3. Cabbage Juice

Cabbage is a vegetable that is low in calories and contains just sixteen calories per serving. Cabbage juice is highly beneficial for people who are looking to lose weight quickly. It helps boost the body's immunity. Regular consumption of cabbage juice will help reduce the risk of developing diabetes as it is rich in vitamin C and anthocyanin. Cabbage juice helps in cutting down your cravings for salty or sugary foods. You can drink it any time before or after meals or even as a snack replacement.

4. Cucumber Juice

This juice is highly effective in reducing weight. Cucumber juice has diuretic properties and helps remove fat and toxins from the body. Cucumber juice helps break down fat from the body and eliminates it through urination. Drinking cucumber juice increases the body's metabolic rate which is important for weight loss. It refreshes the body and gives you a glowing skin and clear complexion. If you are suffering from acidity, heartburn or stomach ulcers, drinking this juice will relieve your symptoms. You can drink cucumber juice before each meal to control your appetite, or you can have it in between meals to keep your stomach feeling full. You can mix some carrots in this juice to make it tastier and healthier.

5. Celery Juice

If you are to shed excess weight, then celery juice is the best option. The overall caloric content is low and helps reduce cellulite formation in the body. It is a diuretic and alleviates puffiness. This juice is rich in fibre and contains vitamins, antioxidants and minerals which are necessary for proper health. It helps control cholesterol level and alleviates digestive problems. This juice is effective in preventing calcification in the body and the formation of stones.

Benefits of Vegetable Juices

- Consuming vegetables in the form of juices will help you take in more vegetables than what a normal person can eat.
- These juices will improve the digestive system by providing a soothing and healing effect.
- As these juices have high levels of dietary fibre, they will aid in weight loss.
- They will help control your hunger pangs and make you feel fuller.
- They are loaded with vitamins, minerals, fibres and antioxidants. This will help in improving your immune system.
- These juices will improve the pH levels of your body and thereby will boost the energy levels of your body.
- These juices will control cholesterol as they do not contain any saturated fats or sodium.
- Drinking vegetable juices three times a day is said to lessen the chance of a person developing Alzheimer's disease.

Chutneys, Papads and Pickles

Chutneys are a ubiquitous part of Indian cuisine. Different varieties of chutneys are prepared and consumed in almost all parts of India. It is not considered a main dish but relished as a condiment. Also, the quantity of chutney served per meal is often small due to its savory nature. The huge popularity of chutney and the Indian diaspora has led to the introduction of chutney in many parts of the world. Mostly, the chutneys are prepared from raw vegetable parts and have the consistency of a paste.

Chutneys can be wet or dry, based on the type. Some of the common flavourings added to them are sugar, salt, garlic, tamarind, ginger and onion. Commonly used spices in chutneys are fenugreek, cumin, coriander, mustard and asafoetida.

Types of Chutney

- **Onion Chutney**

This is a savory chutney usually enjoyed with Indian flat breads. Peeled onions are fried along with garlic flakes, chillies and bengal gram and ground to a paste after adding tamarind and salt. The chutney is then garnished with lightly fried curry leaves and mustard seeds.

- **Mango Chutney**

This is a common chutney enjoyed in the subcontinent. Raw mangoes are sliced into tiny pieces and cooked in water along with slices of garlic and ginger. Afterwards vinegar, chilli pepper, cardamom, sugar, salt and almonds are added to the boiling mixture. After the mixture becomes golden brown and thick, it is cooled and raisins are added to it. If kept in an air-tight jar, it will keep for one week.

- **Yoghurt Chutney**

Fresh green chillies and mint leaves are made into a fine paste after adding salt. This paste is then mixed with yoghurt and beaten well. This simple chutney is best relished with fried food items.

- **Gooseberry Chutney**

This is another easy-to-make chutney. The gooseberries are chopped into small pieces after discarding the seed. The pieces are put in a mixer along with green chillies, coriander leaves and ginger, and made into a fine paste. This chutney is a good source of vitamin C and antioxidants.

- **Date Chutney**

The dates are de-seeded and cooked in water along with ginger, salt, chilli powder, sugar and vinegar, until it thickens. The mixture is then cooled down and raisins and almonds are added to it. After stirring for some time, the chutney is transferred to airtight jars.

- **Coconut Chutney**

This is a commonly found and easily prepared breakfast item. Grated coconut, green chillies, coriander leaves, roasted split peas, yogurt, salt and lime juice are all put in a blender and coarsely ground to a paste.

- **Mint Chutney**

This is a popular chutney found throughout India. Fresh mint leaves along with green chillies, tamarind juice and salt are ground to a paste and served.

- **Tamarind Chutney**

Tamarind is cooked in water for about ten minutes. Tamarind juice is extracted and mixed with molasses, chilli powder, cumin powder and salt. The mixture is heated till it becomes thick and then cooled down before consuming.

- **Peanut Chutney**

De-shelled peanuts are blended with green chillies. Salt, sugar and cumin powder are then added and the mixture is ground to a paste. While serving, it is customary to add lemon juice to the peanut chutney.

- **Garlic Chutney**

Garlic flakes are sautéed along with coconut for some time. These are then ground to a paste with roasted red chillies, tamarind juice and salt.

- **Dried Fish Chutney**

This non-vegetarian chutney comes from the eastern coastal part of India. First, the dried fish are soaked in water for thirty minutes and allowed to dry. The fish are fried till they become golden brown. Grated coconuts, shallots, chopped gingers, red chillies, tamarind, curry leaves and salt are all mixed and fried till they turn brown. All the ingredients are now mixed with the fried fish and ground to a coarse paste.

- **Coriander/Cilantro Chutney**

Cumin and mustard seeds are roasted well and ground to powder. Fresh chopped coriander leaves, chopped onion, coconut pulp, chopped red chillies, lemon juice and salt are mixed with the powdered cumin and mustard seeds. The mixture is then blended to a fine paste to complete the chutney.

Apart from the chutneys described above, there are many varieties prepared from cabbage, curry leaves, guava, radish, tomato, pineapple, fish eggs, shrimp, and so on.

Health Benefits of Chutney

As the ingredients are mostly derived from plants and not cooked, chutneys are usually full of vitamins and other nutrients. Little or no use of oil makes the chutney almost fat-free. Many types of chutney are made sour by adding tamarind, tomato and other sour ingredients. These chutneys are rich in anti-oxidants. The addition of fresh green leaves also ensure abundance of chlorophyll.

A wide variety of chutneys can be made from almost any combination of vegetables, fruits, herbs and spices. Chutneys are usually grouped into sweet or hot forms. Both usually contain spices, including chilli, but differ by their main flavours. Chutney types and their preparations vary widely across the subcontinent.

Types of Chutneys:

Apart from the kinds of chutneys described above, here are some more that are part of Indian cuisine:

- Coriander (cilantro) chutney and mint chutney are often called 'hari chutney', literally 'green chutney'
- Tamarind chutney or imli chutney, often called 'meethi chutney', where meethi means 'sweet' in Hindi
- Sooth or saunth chutney, made with dates and ginger
- Coconut chutney
- Prune chutney
- Lime chutney made from whole, unripe limes.

- Garlic chutney made from fresh garlic, coconut and groundnut
- Green tomato chutney
- Ginger chutney mostly used in Tamil cuisine and Udupi cuisine to be eaten with dosa
- Tomato onion chutney

Some chutneys associated with different parts of the country are:

- Assam: coriander, spinach, tomato, curry leaf, chilli, radish, carrot, cucumber, beetroot, lentil, chickpea, ghost chilli chutneys
- Andhra Pradesh: coconut, coriander, red chilli with gram, tomato, onion, peanut, lemon, curry leaf, tamarind, green chilli, ginger, mint, mango chutneys
- Gujarat: hot lime chutneys, garlic chutney
- Haryana: tamarind chutney
- Himachal Pradesh: guava and eggplant chutneys
- Karnataka: coconut, peanut, tomato, tamarind, mango, urad dal, pudina, heeray kayi (ridge gourd), badane kayi (eggplant), uchellu (niger seed), bende kaayi (okra or ladyfinger), agashi (flax seed), ginger chutneys
- Kerala: coconut, pudina, urad dal, mango, dry fish, shrimp, onion chutney
- Maharashtra: hot raw mango chutney, guramba, panchamrit, mirachicha thecha (dry chutneys made with flaxseed), solapuri shenga, peanut/red chilly powder, karale (niger seed), peanut-garlic, dudhi, roasted bottle gourd skin chutney

- Odisha: coconut, mango, orange, tomato, dried fish chutneys
- Punjab: mint, onion, tamarind, mango chutneys
- Tamil Nadu: coconut, coriander, curry leaf, red chilli, green chilli, tomato, onion, ginger, mint, mango, lentil chutneys.
- Uttar Pradesh and Bihar: coriander seed and leaf, garlic, roasted onion, cooked tomato, mint, radish, amla, sweet and sour mango, green chilly, boiled potato and pickled mango, red chilly and jaggery chutneys.
- West Bengal: lime, green mango, tomato, papaya, pineapple, date, dried mango jelly and other dry fruits, green chilli chutneys.

Pickles and Papad

Pickles often play the role of saviours in Indian meals. They can immediately make any bland or boring food hot and spicy. When you don't like the vegetables or dishes that have been prepared at home, you call for pickle. When the poha or upma seems dry and flavourless, you add some spicy and sour pickle. When there is nothing to eat with parathas, a tablespoon of pickle acts as the best accompaniment. Khichadi in most homes is considered unpalatable unless coupled with some pickle.

Though it is rich in taste, pickle is also one food item which renders healthy stuff unhealthy. Its ingredients, like raw mango, amla, vegetables, lemons, and so on are actually extremely healthy, but the way pickles are made transforms them into being unhealthy and harmful for health.

Like pickles, papad is another favourite side-dish that accompanies most meals. The crisp, multi-flavoured papad has two hidden unhealthy ingredients similar to those found in pickles. However in the case of papad, they do not stand out just as much as they do in pickles.

These two hidden unhealthy ingredients are:

1. **Salt:** A high amount of salt is used in preparing pickles, both for seasoning and preservation. A lot of salt means high sodium intake, which is strongly associated with developing the risk of high blood pressure or hypertension and heart disease. It is recommended that healthy people should consume less than 2,300 mg of sodium or one teaspoon of salt in a day, which you can easily get from your daily food. You actually don't need to add any salt to your diet. Each serving of pickle adds approximately 300 mg of sodium to your daily intake, which is extremely high.

2. **Oil:** It is used as a preservative in addition to imparting taste to pickles. Fruits or vegetables being pickled are chopped and soaked in oil, which protects the pickle from getting moist and spoiling. Oil also prevents contamination of pickles by bacteria and fungi, thereby increasing their shelf-life. However, consuming higher amounts of oil increase your risk of developing cardiac disease.

By saying this, we don't mean you should totally stop treating your taste buds to the spicy and tangy pickles and papads. But you should consider reducing the frequency and quantity of consumption to ensure that you enjoy them, rather than suffer after having them. Opt for homemade pickles and papads where you are sure about the ingredients that have been used. Also, opt for roasted papad instead of fried, to lessen the additional oil that will be used in the frying process.

Conclusion

Now you know what the Great Indian Diet is all about and how it can help you look good and stay healthy. The truth is that it is nothing new. It has been around for thousands of years and it's about time we bring it back into our daily lives. What we know is great, but we need to harness the incredible power of the mind to make all of this work for us in the most effortless way possible. The techniques and tips we have touched upon in this book are part of Indian history and people from all over the world flock to our country to learn it. It's what Shilpa and I use extensively to enhance the quality of our lives, manage stress, and make the process of health and living as meaningful and effortless as possible.

The Importance of Meditation

If there is anything that has added more value to our lives over the last few months, it's the practice of simple meditation. Right from stress to managing emotions effectively, eating healthier, combating cravings to sleeping better and being more mindful about how an exercise or food impacts your mind and body, meditation has guided us in our journey of life.

I used to think meditation is the most difficult thing to do. I guess that's what we make ourselves believe until I really got inspired and actually started 'doing it'.

Regardless of age, health or other factors, regular meditation practice can benefit us profoundly at all levels, even to the innermost reaches of our DNA. Heart health, cellular health and cognitive function have all shown benefits from regular meditation practice. These days an increasing number of medical practitioners recommend this ancient, time-honoured practice. As a result, meditation now holds a well-deserved reputation as a simple, yet powerful and safe practice for supporting health and preventing illness.

It works quickly, and we don't need published studies to tell us that. You can feel the difference yourself even after just ten minutes. Combine this great Indian tradition with the great Indian diet. Start living and stop dieting.

The Power of Gratitude

We would like to end this book by talking about one of the most powerful and inexpensive tools available on this planet—gratitude. All too often, our minds dwell on problems not resolved, opportunities missed, relationships lost, promises not kept, poor health, faded dreams, and fears of an uncertain future, regrets, and longings. While life does bring its share of challenges and disappointments, it also brings us great joy: problems solved, opportunities seized, relationships built, great health, promises kept, dreams fulfilled, hope that reassures our fear—blessing upon blessing. It brings with it the opportunity of today and tomorrow. A clean slate to keep on trying or to start all over again. An opportunity to move forward even an inch each day, in spheres of our life such as health, wealth, career, relationships and spirituality. An opportunity to be a little bit better than what we were yesterday. An opportunity to practise kindness and cut down on worry.

Gratitude is a thankful appreciation for what an individual receives, whether tangible or intangible. With gratitude, people acknowledge the goodness in their lives. In the process, people usually recognize that the source of that goodness lies at least partially outside themselves. As a result, gratitude also helps people connect to something larger than themselves as individuals—whether to other people, nature, or a higher power.

We have seen the power of gratitude transform the health of extremely sick people. We have seen victims of cancer turn their lives around by changing the way they think, by changing their attitudes towards life and all around. We have seen people throw away their sleeping pills and anxiety medicines because they learnt it was never a cure, and the real cure lay in their minds, in their attitudes and outlook towards life and themselves. We have seen gratitude transform relationships and careers and how it has inspired people who would never work out or eat well, to start doing so.

In positive psychology research, gratitude is strongly and consistently associated with greater happiness. Gratitude helps people feel more positive emotions, relish good experiences, improve their health, deal with adversity, and build strong relationships. People feel and express gratitude in multiple ways. They can apply it to the past (retrieving positive memories and being thankful for elements of childhood or past blessings), the present (not taking good fortune for granted as it comes), and the future (maintaining a hopeful and optimistic attitude). Regardless of the inherent or current level of someone's gratitude, it's a quality that individuals can successfully cultivate further.

You can find ways to give thanks for all that you have and all that you are. Spend less time counting calories and more time counting your blessings. Don't compare yourself with other people or design your behaviour, lifestyle, and self to be what other people want. That may be your biggest misery. Stay real and be who you are meant to be. Take each day as it comes, giving thanks for the little things in your life, and remember that it is the sum of small things that make up the bigger beautiful picture.

Tips on how to cultivate gratitude in your life

- *Write a thank-you note:* You can make yourself happier and nurture your relationship with another person by writing a thank-you letter expressing your enjoyment and appreciation of that person's impact on your life. Send it, or better yet, deliver and read it in person if possible. Make a habit of sending at least one gratitude letter a month.

- *Thank someone mentally:* No time to write? It may help just to think about someone who has done something nice for you, and mentally thank the individual.

- *Keep a gratitude journal:* Make it a habit to write down or share with a loved one thoughts about the gifts you've received each day.

- *Count your blessings:* Pick a time every week to sit down and write about your blessings — reflecting on what went right or what you are grateful for. Sometimes it helps to pick a number — such as three to five things — that you will identify each week. As you write, be specific and think about the sensations you felt when something good happened to you.

- *Pray:* People who are religious can use prayer to cultivate gratitude.

- *Meditate:* Mindfulness meditation involves focusing on the present moment without judgement. Although people often focus on a word or phrase (such as 'peace'), it is also possible to focus on what you're grateful for (the warmth of the sun, a pleasant sound, etc.).

Gratitude is a way for people to appreciate what they have instead of always reaching out for something new in the hope that it will make them happier, or thinking that they can't feel satisfied until every physical and material need is met. Gratitude helps people refocus on what they have instead of what they lack. And, although it may feel contrived at first, this mental state grows stronger with use and practice.

We hope you enjoyed reading the book and will take back ways to enrich it. The great Indian diet is our gift to all our fans, followers and readers who would like to join us on this journey of a healthier and happier life.

Acknowledgements

To Viaan Raj, my son. Motherhood made me realize the value of life and drove me to write this book for mothers who need help but don't know who to ask. Good food choices are the reason for good health. That should be paramount and cannot be taken for granted.

To Ma, for inculcating in me the right habits and choices, in food and in life. For selflessly cooking for us, teaching us the value of food, not just nutritionally but also as a means of bringing the family together at mealtimes. The greatest meals are those prepared with love, and yours was unconditional. Thank you for this life, your blessings, your strength, and much more.

To Dad, for your work ethics and discipline, and above all for being supportive always. Through your actions, you showed me the respect and love women deserve, as well as the value of discipline if one is a foodie. (At seventy-four, he walks and does yoga almost every day.)

To my sister, Shamita. No one knows this secret. I grew interested in food and nutrition only because of you and your obsession with losing weight seventeen years ago, when you were reading *Fit for Life*. It was you who first told me the difference between 'proteins' and 'carbs'. Thus began my journey to discovering food. You are a rockstar, my Tunki.

To Luke Coutinho, for your immense knowledge and faith. This book has been a learning curve even for me. I am so glad we met and shared the same passion. Simplifying and debunking so many myths related to Indian food would have been an uphill task if not for you.

To Aksha Tanna, my Gemini twin, thank you for telling me about Luke Coutinho. You cannot imagine how valuable that introduction has been.

To Anishi, my brand (rather 'life') manager, for being the best friend ever to me and 'bad cop' for others. You play both roles to perfection. Thanks also to the entire Team Exceed.

To my father-in- law, for willingly being my first scapegoat. He followed the 'Great Indian Diet' diligently and reiterated my faith in it, especially since he lost 13 kilos in two and a half months. Love you, Dad.

To Milee, Caroline, and everyone at Penguin Random House, for believing in this book.

I saved the best for the last.

To Raj, my husband. If my parents made me believe that anything is possible, you made it possible for me to achieve even the impossible. You've played catalyst in many of my entrepreneurial ventures, even the introduction to my publisher. And thank you for eating whatever you are served at the table, even if you don't like it! You are the wind beneath my wings, my soulmate, my hero forever.

Shilpa Shetty Kundra

* * *

To Natashya Phillips Coutinho—Thank you for your immense support and encouragement in making this dream and book come true. For putting up with my changing moods, late nights away from home spent at coffee shops writing, the travel to do what I love doing. All this, especially when Tyanna was just born, and I couldn't be around as much as I should have.

To Tyanna Brooklyn Coutinho—You were in your mommy's womb when Shilpa and I began this journey. From then till now, you've been the most amazing gift I could ever have been given. From the time you ate your first raw garlic at four months, curry leaves, carrots and broccoli, and biting of bits of papaya leaf with Daddy from our plants in Goa, till the time you did your first set of squats and your first downward dog, it's been a magical journey that will continue for the rest of your life. This book is for you. You are beautiful and will always be so.

To my family—Too large to mention, but every one of you is a massive motivation and inspiration in my life. When I reminisce about my days as a child until now, the journey has been diverse and magical. Unconditional love always, to each and every one of you, forever.

The different energies I have experienced over the last two years that have changed the way I live and think, energies that challenged the '3-D' of life, energies that cause bliss, peace, happiness, confusion, anger, sadness and longing, haunting and yet ecstatically blissful energies that have evoked a certain wisdom in me, and constantly remind me about the beauty, mysteriousness, and uncertainty of life, love and inner peace. Priceless!

To Shilpa—We connected on a different level for a reason that may seem larger than life, giving back to the world with the intention to change health and lifestyle, reduce suffering and pain. It's been an amazing journey with you. Your humility and realness have inspired me the most. Every moment spent with you has been enriching and so much fun.

To my GOQii team—For the immense support as always, and managing without me when I needed (and will need) to be away. Vishal Gondal, for your understanding, inspiration and compassion, thank you.

Special thanks to Vrushali Athavale, Hardika Vira, Sneha, Shimpli—four of my best nutritionists and lifestyle coaches, for their valuable inputs, suggestions and incredible support. You helped fill valuable gaps.

Thank you, Milee, for truly being such a massive support through this process. You have been so flexible and available right through, and I think this book would not have been possible without your help and understanding.

Thank you, Amulya and Vani Aunty, for getting me into the practice of yoga and meditation. It has been life-changing , and pranayama and meditation are probably the most prescribed 'drugs' on my prescriptions to my patients and clients worldwide.

Luke Coutinho

Note on the Authors

Shilpa Shetty Kundra is a popular Bollywood actor, model, entrepreneur and health enthusiast. A yoga believer, she produced a yoga DVD, and was first amongst actors making yoga 'cool'. Since making her debut in the film *Baazigar*, she has appeared in nearly sixty Bollywood, Tamil, Telugu and Kannada films. Shilpa is the recipient of numerous awards and nominations, including four nominations at the Filmfare Awards.

Shilpa is also Chairman of Best Deal TV, India's first celebrity home shopping channel, and IOSIS spa and salons that have seventeen centres across India.

Shilpa is the winner of the international reality television series, 'Celebrity Big Brother 5', which catapulted her to fame. She featured as a celebrity host for the 2008 reality show, 'Bigg Boss 2', and served as a talent judge for the reality shows, 'Jhalak Dikhla Jaa' (season 1) and 'Nach Baliye' (seasons 5 and 6). Shetty turned into a film producer with the 2014 action film, 'Dishkiyaaoon'. She has always been a trendsetter, whether it be fashion or ideas, even designing her own line of sarees under the 'SSK' brand.

She lives in Mumbai with her husband, Raj, and her son Viaan-Raj. This is her debut book, co-authored with Luke Coutinho

Luke Coutinho is a holistic nutritionist, speaker, and exercise physiologist, lifestyle medicine and integrative healer. Benchmarked in the top ten leading nutritionists across India and one of the top ten personal trainers across the country, Luke is also an international collaborator with Yale–Griffin, Research and Prevention Centre, C.T, U.S.A. training partner, Nutrition Detectives. Luke has been involved in nutrition, coaching and fitness ever since he graduated from IHM with specialization in food science and nutrition. He works with obesity, disease, lifestyle and children across the world. Luke currently specializes in cancer and handles cases across the globe. His clientele is globally placed across New York, Belgium, Singapore, Hong Kong, Dubai, and India. He also consults with several celebrities across various industries including Bollywood.

Luke is the founder and director of Herbs Nutrition Pvt. Ltd. He is also the head nutritionist, master coach and mastermind behind GOQii's lifestyle and health coaching model. Luke is also the author of *Eat Smart, Move More, Sleep Right–Your Personal Health Coach*. This is his second book.